Basic Toxicology

Basic Toxicology
Fundamentals, Target Organs, and Risk Assessment

Frank C. Lu

Consulting Toxicologist
Miami, Florida

⬤ HEMISPHERE PUBLISHING CORPORATION, Washington
A subsidiary of Harper & Row, Publishers, Inc.

Cambridge   Philadelphia   San Francisco   Washington
London   Mexico City   São Paulo   Singapore   Sydney

This book was set in Press Roman by Hemisphere Publishing Corporation.
The editors were Roberta Robey and Sandra J. King; the cover designer was
Susan Mohamed; the production supervisor was Miriam Gonzalez; and the
typesetter was Wayne Hutchins.
Braun-Brumfield, Inc. was printer and binder.

BASIC TOXICOLOGY: Fundamentals, Target Organs, and Risk Assessment

5 6 7 8 9 0   B R B R   8 9 8 7

Library of Congress Cataloging in Publication Data

Lu, Frank C.
  Basic toxicology.

  Includes bibliographies and index.
  1. Toxicology. I. Title. [DNLM: 1. Poisons.
2. Toxicology—methods. QV 602 L926b]
RA1211.L8   1985   615.9   84-12761
ISBN 0-89116-389-1 (hard cover)
ISBN 0-89116-468-5 (soft cover)

Contents

PART III TARGET ORGANS

Preface

Toxicology is an important science. It provides a sound basis for formulating measures to protect the health of workers against toxicants in factories, farms, mines, and other occupational environments. It is also valuable in the protection of public health against hazards associated with toxic substances in food, air, and water. Toxicology has played and will continue to play a significant role in the health and welfare of the world.

Cognizant of the importance of toxicology, WHO organized a toxicology training course in China in 1982, as part of the ongoing China–WHO collaborative program on medical sciences. The course consisted of two parts. The author was invited to lecture on basic toxicology, whereas lectures on occupational toxicology were given by others. This book originated from the author's lecture notes.

The subjects covered in the book are divided into three parts; they are general principles, testing procedures, and target organs. The first part deals with absorption, distribution, and excretion of toxicants; their biotransformation (detoxication and bioactivation); their adverse effects; and factors that modify their effects. It also includes chapters dealing with various approaches to toxicologic evaluation, including risk assessent, and the type and amount of data required to carry out such evaluations.

Part II covers topics related to conventional toxicity studies of different durations. It also deals with the nature of and tests for such specific effects as carcinogenesis, mutagenesis, and teratogenesis. Part III deals with toxic effects on specific target organs: the respiratory system, liver, kidney, skin, eye, nervous system, and a number of others. The effects of toxicants are not described systematically, but they are used in illustrating various categories of toxic effects and the underlying mode of action. Knowledge of general toxicology in its diverse field will promote better understanding of toxicologic data on specific toxic substances and their interactions.

This book is intended as an introductory text for students taking toxicology courses and for those involved in allied sciences who require a background in toxicology. Furthermore, since toxicology is a vast subject and is fast expanding, the book is likely to be useful to those who have become specialized in one or a few areas in toxicology but wish to brush-up in other areas.

In preparing this book, attempts were made to have a relatively comprehensive coverage of the subjects as well as to maintain brevity. The latter was achieved by the inclusion of some appendices and a large number of references to assist readers interested in additional information.

Part One

General Principles of Toxicology

Chapter 1

General Considerations

People are exposed to a great variety of natural and man-made substances. Under certain conditions such exposures cause adverse health effects, ranging in severity from death to subtle biologic changes. Society's ever-increasing desire to identify and prevent these effects has prompted the dramatic evolution of toxicology as a study of poisons to the present-day complex science.

DEFINITION AND PURPOSE OF TOXICOLOGY

To state it simply and concisely, toxicology is the study of the nature and mechanism of toxic effects of substances on living organisms and other biologic systems. It also deals with quantitative assessment of the severity and frequency of these effects in relation to the exposure of the organisms.

The assessment of health hazards of industrial chemicals, environmental pollutants, and other substances represents an important element in the protection of the health of the worker and members of communities. In-depth studies of the nature and mechanism of the effects of toxicants are invaluable in the invention of specific antidotes and other ameliorative measures. Along with other sciences, toxicology contributes to the development of safer chemicals used as drugs, food additives, and pesticides. The toxic effects per se are exploited in the pursuit of more effective insecticides, anthelmintics, antimicrobials, and agents used in chemical warfare.

SCOPE

Toxicology has a broad scope. It deals with toxicity studies of chemicals used (1) in medicine for diagnostic, preventive, and therapeutic purposes, (2) in food industry as direct and indirect additives, (3) in agriculture as pesticides, growth regulators, artificial pollinators, and animal feed additives, and (4) in chemical industry as solvents, components, and intermediates of plastics and many other types of chemicals. It is also concerned with the health effects of metals (as in mines and smelters), petroleum products, paper and pulp, toxic plants, and animal toxins.

EARLY DEVELOPMENT

The earliest human was well aware of the toxic effects of a number of substances, such as venoms of snakes, the poisonous plants hemlock and aconite, and the toxic mineral substances arsenic, lead, and antimony. Some of these were actually used intentionally for their toxic effects to commit homicide and suicide. For centuries, homicides with toxic substances were not uncommon in Europe. To protect against poisoning, there were continual efforts directed toward the discovery and development of preventive and antidotal measures. However, a more critical evaluation of these measures was only begun by Maimonides (1135-1204) with his famous *Poisons and Their Antidotes*, published in 1198.

More significant contributions to the evolution of toxicology were made in the 16th century and later. Paracelsus stated: "No substance is a poison by itself. It is the dose that makes a substance a poison" and "the right dose differentiates a poison and a remedy." These statements laid the foundation of the concept of the "dose-response relation" and the "therapeutic index" developed later. In addition, he described in his book *Bergsucht* (1533-1534) the clinical manifestations of chronic arsenic and mercury poisoning as well as miner's disease. This might be considered the forefather of occupational toxicology. Orfila wrote an important treatise (1814-1815) describing a systematic correlation between the chemical and biologic information on certain poisons. He also devised methods for detecting poisons and pointed to the necessity for chemical analysis for legal proof of lethal intoxication. The introduction of this approach ushered in a speciality area of modern toxicology, namely, forensic toxicology. References to these and a number of later developments are given by Casarett and Bruce (1980).

RECENT DEVELOPMENTS

In the face of a growing population, modern society demands improvements of the health and living conditions, including nutrition, clothing, dwelling, and transportation. To meet this goal, a great variety of chemicals, many of them in large quantities, must be manufactured and used. It has been estimated that tens of thousands of different chemicals are in commercial production in industrialized countries. In one way or another, these chemicals come in contact with various segments of the population: people are engaged in their manufacture, handling, use (e.g., painters, applicators of pesticides), consumption (e.g., drugs, food additives), or misuse (e.g., suicide, accidental poisoning). Furthermore, people may be exposed to the more persistent chemicals via various environmental media.

There is, therefore, a need to render the task of toxicologically assessing the vast number of chemicals more manageable. As an attempt to fulfill this need, criteria have been proposed and adopted for the selection of chemicals to be tested according to their priority. In addition, the "tier systems" allow decisions to be made at different stages of toxicologic testing, thus avoiding unnecessary studies. This procedure has been particularly useful in the testing for carcinogenicity, mutagenicity, and immunotoxicity because of the large expenses involved and the great multitude of test systems that are available (Chapters 6, 9, 10, and 18).

Because of the large number of people exposed to these chemicals, society cannot defer appropriate control until serious injuries have appeared. The modern toxicologist, therefore, must attempt to identify, where possible, indicators of exposure and early, reversible signs of health effects. These will permit the formulation of decisions at the right time to safeguard the health of individuals, either as occupational workers or in exposed communities. The achievements in these areas have assisted responsible personnel in instituting appropriate medical surveillance of occupational workers and other exposed populations. Notable examples are the use of cholinesterase inhibition as an indicator of exposure to organophosphorous pesticides and a variety of biochemical parameters to monitor for lead exposure.

Advances made in biochemical and chemobiokinetic studies, as well as those in genetic toxicology, immunotoxicology, and morphologic studies on a subcellular level, have all contributed to a better understanding of the nature, site, and mechanism of action of toxicants. For example, technological breakthroughs enabled in vitro studies to demonstrate that whether the hepatocytes or the nonparenchymal cells are affected by a chemical carcinogen is related to differences in their ability to repair the DNA damage induced by the chemical (Lewis and Swenberg, 1980). Numerous studies have shown that the responses to toxicants are better correlated with the effective dose, i.e., the concentration of the toxicant at the site of action, rather than the administered dose. Furthermore, where the effect results mainly or entirely from an active metabolite, the concentration of the metabolite rather than that of the parent chemical is important.

To translate scientific knowledge into basic tools for the health profession, the toxicologist is ever more involved in the determination of safe exposure limits or an assessment of the risks. The former includes the "acceptable daily intakes" (WHO, 1962) and the "threshold limit values" (Federal Register, 1971), whereas the latter is used in connection with substances the effects of which are believed to have no threshold or their threshold cannot be determined.

These determinations involve comprehensive studies of the toxic properties, demonstration of dosages that produce no observable adverse effects, establishment of dose-effect and dose-response relationships, and chemobiokinetic and biotransformation studies.

SOME CHALLENGES AND SUCCESSES

The so-called aniline tumors were reported by Rehn (1895), a German surgeon, in the urinary bladder of three men who had worked in an aniline factory. The role of aniline and aniline dyes was confirmed only some 40 years later, after much experimental investigation in animals (e.g., Hueper and co-workers, 1938) and extensive epidemiologic studies by Case et al. (1954) had been carried out. This discovery led to improved occupational standards and more stringent controls of food colors derived from coal tar.

In the late 1950s, thalidomide was widely used as a sedative. It has a very low acute toxicity and readily met the toxicity testing protocol prevailing at that time. However, a rare form of congenital malformation, phocomelia (the virtual absence of extremities), was observed among some offspring of mothers who had taken this drug during the first trimester (Lenz and Knapp, 1962). This tragedy led to the explosive development of teratology, an important specialty area of toxicology.

The once prevalent lead poisoning in certain areas of industrialized countries has now largely disappeared. This great accomplishment in the field of public health resulted from the implementation of control measures devised on the basis of the knowledge gained from the numerous toxicologic studies of lead.

Many cases of serious illness that culminate in permanent paralysis and death have been reported in Minamata and Niigata in Japan in the 1950s and 1960s, respectively (Study Group of Minamata Disease, 1968; Tsubaki and Irukayama, 1977). The cause of the illness was eventually traced to methyl mercury in the fish caught locally. The fish was contaminated with this chemical, which had been discharged as such into the water by a factory, or the contaminant was derived from elemental mercury discharged by the factory and methylated through certain microorganisms in the mud. Measures to rehabilitate the surviving patients and legal control of the factors have been instituted.

On the other hand, the cause of another mysterious illness in Japan, known as itai-itai disease, remains unsolved, although cadmium apparently played a role. The patients had resided for many years in areas that were in the vicinity of mines and where the cadmium levels in rice and water were excessive.

A more solid foundation in the assessment of risks of chemical carcinogens resulted from recent advances in epidemiologic studies, carcinogenic bioassays, short-term mutagenesis/carcinogenesis tests, studies on carcinogen-DNA adduct, chemobiokinetics, and biometrics, as well as the realization that carcinogens differ in their potency, mode of action, and latency (Chapter 7).

FUTURE PROSPECTS

Along with future modernization, it is inevitable that food from new, unconventional sources, which require very little land compared to conventional farming, will be relied on to augment our food supply. The safety of such foods will require appropriate safety evaluation.

Toxicology can provide, in conjunction with other sciences, safer alternative chemicals for agricultural, industrial, and consumer uses through the determination of structure-toxicity relationships. A reduction of toxicity may be achieved by altering the target toxicity or by changing the chemobiokinetics. The value and limitations of this approach have been discussed (Goldberg, 1983).

Some recent breakthroughs in other fields of science and technology will enable the development of new drugs to treat diseases that are now incurable. It has been estimated that petroleum, which provides many of our necessities, will run short in 10-20 years. In anticipation of this predicament, efforts to develop synfuels will shift to high gear in the foreseeable future. These and many other modernization schemes will undoubtedly require the development and use of many new chemicals. Assessment of their safety will be the challenge and responsibility of the toxicologist.

In response to a societal call, on humane grounds, to reduce the use of laboratory animals, isolated organs, cultured tissues, cells, and lower forms of life will be increasingly used. Such test systems will likely be faster and cheaper, and will augment the variety of studies, especially those related to the mechanism of toxicity.

Because of the increasing demand on the limited facilities for toxicologic testing and on the short supply of qualified personnel, it is of utmost importance that toxicity data generated anywhere be accepted internationally. However, to ensure general acceptance, the data must meet certain prerequisites. The "Good Laboratory Practice" promulgated by the U.S. Food and Drug Administration (FDA, 1980) represents a useful step in the right direction.

Finally, toxicologists must continue to improve testing procedures to reduce the proportions of false-positive and false-negative results and to conduct studies designed to promote better understanding of the significance of toxic effects in order to achieve more satisfactory assessment of the safety/risk of toxicants.

REFERENCES

Casarett, L. J., and Bruce, M. C. (1980) Origin and scope of toxicology. In: *Casarett and Doull's Toxicology*. Eds. J. Doull, C. D. Klaassen and M. O. Amdur. New York: Macmillan.

Case, R. A. M., Hosker, M. E., McDonald, D. B., and Pearson, J. T. (1954) Tumours of the urinary bladder in workmen engaged in the manufacture and use of certain dyestuff intermediates in the British chemical industry, *Br. J. Ind. Med.* 11:75–104.

Federal Register (1971) *Threshold Limit Values adopted by the American Conference of Governmental Industrial Hygienists, 1968.* Vol. 36, No. 105, May 29. Washington, D.C.: U.S. Government Printing Office.

Golberg, L. (1983) *Structure-Activity Correlation as a Predictive Tool in Toxicology*. Washington, D.C.: Hemisphere.

Hueper, W. C., et al. (1938) Experimental production of bladder tumors in dogs by administration of beta-napthylamine. *J. Ind. Hyg. Toxicol.* 20:46.

Lenz, W., and Knapp, K. (1962) Thalidomide embryopathy. *Arch. Environ. Health* 5:100–105.

Lewis, J. G., and Swenberg, J. A. (1980) Differential repair of O^6-methyl guanine in DNA of rat hepatocytes and nonparenchymal cells. *Nature* 288: 185–187.

Rehn, L. (1895) Blasengeschwulste bei Fuchsin-Arbeiten. *Arch. Klin. Chir.* 50:588.

Study Group on Minamata Disease (1968) *Minamata Disease*. Minamata, Japan: Minamata University.

Tsubaki, T. and Irukayama, K. (1977) *Minamata Disease: Methyl Mercury Poisoning in Minamata and Niigata, Japan*. New York: Elsevier Scientific.

WHO (1962) Sixth Report of the Joint FAD/WHO Expert Committee on Food Additives. Geneva: World Health Organization.

ADDITIONAL READING

FDA (1980) Code of Federal Regulations, Title 21, Food and Drugs. Part 58. Washington, D.C.: U.S. Government Printing Office.

Chapter 2

Absorption, Distribution, and Excretion of Toxicants

INTRODUCTION

Apart from local effects at the site of contact, a toxicant can cause injury only after it is absorbed by the organism. Absorption can occur through the skin, the gastrointestinal tract, the lungs, and several minor routes. Furthermore, the nature and intensity of the effects of a chemical on an organism depend on its concentration in the target organs. The concentration depends not only on the administered dose but also on other factors, including absorption, distribution, binding, and excretion. For a chemical to be absorbed, distributed, and eventually excreted, a toxicant must pass through a number of cell membranes. A cell membrane generally consists of a biomolecular layer of lipid molecules with proteins scattered throughout the membrane (see Fig. 2-1).

There are four mechanisms by which a toxicant may pass through a cell membrane; the most important of them is passive diffusion through the membrane. The others are filtration through the membrane pores, carrier-mediated transport, and engulfing by the cell. The last two mechanisms are different in that the cell takes an active part in the transfer of a toxicant across its membranes.

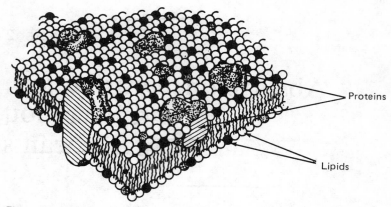

Figure 2-1 Schematic diagram of biologic membrane. Spheres represent head groups (phosphatidylcholine), and zig-zag lines indicate tail ends of lipids. Black, white, and stippled spheres indicate different kinds of lipids. Large bodies represent proteins; some are located on the surface, others within the membrane. (Modified from S. J. Singer and G. L. Nicholson, *Science*, 175:720. By permission of the author and the American Association for the Advancement of Science, copyright © 1972.)

Passive Diffusion

Most toxicants cross cell membranes by simple, passive diffusion. The rate of passage is related directly to the concentration gradient across the membrane, and to the lipid solubility. For example, mannitol is hardly absorbed (< 2%); acetylsalicylic acid is fairly well absorbed (21%); and thiopental is even more readily absorbed (67%). It is noteworthy that the chloroform:water partition of the nonionized forms of these chemicals are, respectively, < 0.002, 2.0, and 100. For references to this and other examples see Timbrell (1982).

Many toxicants are ionizable. The ionized form is often unable to penetrate the cell membrane because of its low lipid solubility. On the other hand, the nonionized form is likely lipid-soluble enough to do so, and its rate of penetration is dependent on the lipid solubility. The extent of ionization of weak organic acids and bases depends on the pH of the medium. Thus, for the former, such as benzoic acid, diffusion is facilitated in acidic environment, where they exist mainly in the nonionized form; for the latter, such as aniline, diffusion is facilitated in basic environment.

Filtration

The membranes of the capillaries and the glomeruli have relatively large pores (about 40 Å) and allow molecules smaller than albumin (molecular weight 60,000) to pass through. Bulk flow of water through these pores results from hydrostatic and/or osmotic pressure and can act as carrier of toxicants. The pores in most cells, however, are relatively small (about 4 Å) and allow chemicals only up to a molecular weight of 100–200 to pass through. Chemicals of larger molecules, therefore, can filter into and out of the capillaries. They can, therefore, establish equilibrium between the concentrations in the plasma and in the extracellular fluid, but they cannot do so by filtration between the extracellular and intracellular fluids.

Carrier-Mediated Transport

This involves the formation of a complex between the chemical and a macromolecular carrier on one side of the membrane. The complex then diffuses to the other side of the membrane, where the chemical is released. Thereafter the carrier returns to the original surface to repeat the transport process. The carrier has a limited capacity. When it is saturated, the rate of transport is no longer dependent on the concentration of the chemical and assumes zero order kinetics. Structure, conformation, size, and charge are important in determining the affinity of a chemical for a carrier site, and competitive inhibition can occur among chemicals with similar characteristics.

Active transport involves a carrier that moves molecules across a membrane against a concentration gradient, or, if the molecule is an ion, against an electrochemical gradient. It requires the expenditures of metabolic energy and can be inhibited by poisons that interfere with cell metabolism.

Facilitated diffusion is similar to active transport but does not move molecules against a concentration gradient. Furthermore, it is not energy-dependent, and metabolic poisons will not inhibit this process.

Engulfing by the Cell

Particles may be engulfed by cells. When the particles are solid, the process is called phagocytosis and when they are liquid, it is called pinocytosis. Such special transport systems are important for removal of particulate matter from the alveoli and of certain toxic substances from the blood by the reticuloendothelial system. Absorption of carrageenans (mol. wt. about 40,000) from the gut is also by this process.

ABSORPTION

The main routes by which toxicants are absorbed are the gastrointestinal tract, lungs, and skin. However, in toxicologic studies, such special routes as intraperitoneal, intramuscular, and subcutaneous injections are often used.

Gastrointestinal Tract

Many toxicants can enter the GI tract along with food and water or alone as drugs or other types of chemicals. With the exception of those that are caustic or very irritating to the mucosa, most toxicants do not exert any toxic effect unless they are absorbed. Absorption can take place along the entire GI tract. For example, certain drugs are administered as sublingual tablets and supposi- tories to be absorbed in the mouth and the rectum, respectively. However, the mouth and rectum are, in general, insignificant sites of absorption of environ- mental chemicals.

The stomach is a significant site of absorption, especially for weak acids, which will exist in the diffusible, nonionized, lipid-soluble form. On the other hand, weak bases will be highly ionized in the acidic gastric juice and therefore not generally absorbable. Absorption from the intestine is also mainly by diffu- sion. Because of their near neutral pH, both weak bases and weak acids are in the nonionized, diffusible form and hence readily absorbable.

Figure 2-2 shows benzoic acid, which is a weak acid, exists in the stomach mainly in the nonionized form, and is thus readily absorbed. Aniline, a weak base, existing mainly in the ionized form, is poorly absorbed. In the small intestine, the reverse is true (Fig. 2-3). The circulating plasma, which is slightly alkaline, facilitates the absorption of benzoic acid by removing the ionized form. While favoring the nonionized form of aniline, the plasma nevertheless also facilitates the absorption from the stomach and the intestine by removing the ionized form through circulation and distribution of the chemical.

In the intestine, there are special carrier-mediated transport systems that are responsible for the absorption of nutrients, e.g., monosaccharides, amino acids, and such elements as iron, calcium, and sodium. However, a few toxicants, e.g., 5-fluorouracil, thallium, and lead, are known to be absorbable from the intestine by active transport systems. In addition, particulate matters such as those of the azo dyes and polystyrene latex can enter the intestinal cell by pinocytosis.

Respiratory Tract

The main site of absorption in the respiratory tract is the alveoli in the lungs. This is especially true for gases such as carbon monoxide, nitrogen oxides, and sulfur dioxide and for vapors of volatile liquids such as benzene and carbon tetrachloride. Their ready absorption is related to the large alveolar area, high blood flow, and proximity of the blood to the alveolar air.

The rate of absorption, however, is dependent on the solubility of the gas in the blood, where solubility is defined as the ratio of the concentration of dissolved gas in fluid (blood) to the concentration in the gaseous phase. On the other hand, equilibrium between the blood and the air is reached more quickly for relatively insoluble chemicals, such as ethylene, compared to more soluble chemicals, such as chloroform. In the latter case, absorption is limited by the respiratory volume. If the chemical also has a high solubility in tissues (e.g., fat), even more time will be required to reach equilibrium.

In addition to gases, liquid aerosols will pass through the alveolar cell

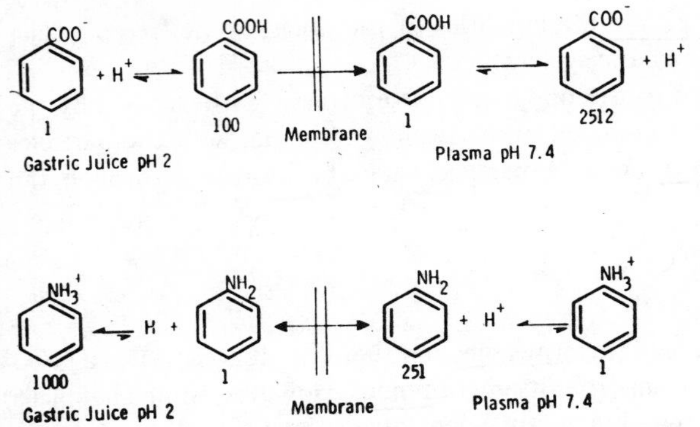

Figure 2-2 Disposition of benzoic acid and aniline in gastric juice and plasma. Figures immediately below the structural formulas represent proportions of ionized and nonionized forms (from Timbrell, 1982, p. 29).

membranes by passive diffusion. Airborne particles vary greatly in size. The sizes of interest from a biologic standpoint range from about 0.1 to 10 μm. Larger particles do not usually enter the respiratory tract; when they do, they are deposited in the nose and disposed of by wiping, blowing, and sneezing. A detailed examination of the percent retention of inhaled aerosol particles in various parts of the human respiratory tract has been provided by Hatch and Gross (1964). However, as a rough estimate, 25% of inhaled particles are exhaled, 50% are deposited in the upper respiratory tract, and 25% are deposited in the lower respiratory tract (Morrow et al., 1966).

Minute particulate matter (less than 1 μm) is either aspirated onto the mucociliary escalator of the tracheobronchial region or engulfed by phagocytes. These phagocytes will then either migrate to the distal end of the mucociliary

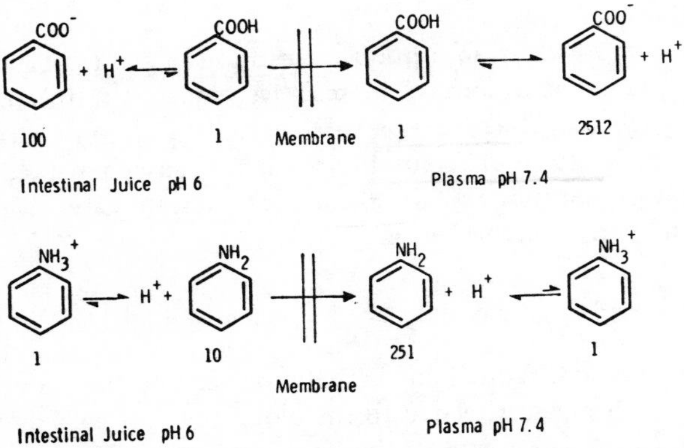

Figure 2-3 Disposition of benzoic acid and aniline in intestinal juice and plasma (from Timbrell, 1982, p. 30).

escalator or be absorbed into the lymphatics of the lungs. Some free particles can also migrate via the lymphatic system.

The particles deposited in the upper respiratory tract may be carried by the cilia to the pharynx and be coughed up or swallowed, along with the particles inhaled through the mouth. Soluble particles may be absorbed through the epithelium into the blood.

Skin

In general, the skin is relatively impermeable, and therefore it constitutes a good barrier, separating the organism from its environment. However, some chemicals can be absorbed through the skin in sufficient quantities to produce systemic effects.

A chemical may be absorbed via the hair follicles or through the cells of the sweat glands or those of the sebaceous glands. These are, however, minor routes for absorption since they constitute only a small surface area of the skin. Therefore, the percutaneous absorption of a chemical is essentially through the skin proper, which consists of the epidermis and dermis.

The first phase of percutaneous absorption is diffusion of the toxicant through the epidermis, which, especially its stratum corneum, is the most important barrier. The stratum corneum consists of several layers of thin, cohesive, dead cells that contain chemically resistant material (protein filament). Small amounts of polar substances appear to diffuse through the outer surface of the protein filaments of the hydrated stratum corneum; nonpolar substances dissolve in and diffuse through the lipid matrix between the protein filaments.

In the human stratum corneum, there are significant differences in structure and chemistry from one region of the body to another, which are reflected in the permeability to chemicals. For example, toxicants cross the scrotum readily, cross the abdominal skin less readily, and cross the sole and palm with great difficulty (Zbinden, 1976).

The second phase of percutaneous absorption is diffusion of the toxicant through the dermis, which contains a porous, nonselective, aqueous diffusion medium. Therefore it is much less effective as a barrier than the stratum corneum, and, as a consequence, abrasion or removal of the latter causes a marked increase in the percutaneous absorption. Acids, alkalis, and mustard gases will also increase the absorption by injuring this barrier.

DISTRIBUTION

After a chemical enters the blood, it is distributed rapidly throughout the body. The rate of distribution to each organ is related to the blood flow through the organ, the ease with which the chemical crosses the local capillary wall and the cell membrane, and the affinity of components of the organ for the chemical.

Barriers

The *blood-brain barrier* is located at the capillary wall. The capillary endothelial cells there are tightly joined, leaving few or no pores between these cells (Bradbury, 1984). Thus, the toxicant has to pass through the capillary endothelium itself. A lack of vesicles in these cells further reduces their transport ability. Finally, the protein concentration of the interstitial fluid in the brain is low, in contrast to that in other organs; protein binding therefore does not serve as a mechanism for the transfer of toxicants from the blood to the brain. For these reasons, the penetration of toxicants into the brain is dependent on their lipid solubility. An outstanding example is the toxicant methyl mercury, which enters the brain readily and the main toxicity of which is on the central nervous system. In contrast, inorganic mercury compounds are not lipid-soluble, do not enter the brain readily, and exert their main adverse effects not on the brain but on the kidney.

The *placental barrier* differs anatomically among various animal species. There are six layers of cells between fetal and maternal blood in some species, whereas in others there is only one layer. Furthermore, the number of layers may change as the gestation progresses. Although the relationship of the number of layers of the placenta to its permeability needs quantitative determination, the placental barrier does impede the transfer of toxicants to the fetus, which is therefore protected to some extent. However, the concentration of a toxicant such as methyl mercury may be higher in certain fetal organs, such as the brain, because of the less effective fetal blood-brain barrier. On the other hand, the fetal concentration of the food coloring amaranth is only 0.03–0.06% of that of the mother (Munro and Willes, 1978).

Other barriers are also present in such organs as the eyes and testicles. In addition, the erythrocyte plays an interesting role in the distribution of certain toxicants. For example, its membrane acts as a barrier against the penetration of inorganic mercury compounds but not that of alkyl mercury. Furthermore, there is affinity of the erythrocyte cytoplasm for alkyl mercury compounds. Because of these factors, the concentration of inorganic mercury compounds in the erythrocytes is only about half that in the plasma, whereas that of methyl mercury in the erythrocyte is about ten times that in the plasma.

Binding and Storage

As noted above, binding of a chemical in a tissue can result in a higher concentration in that tissue. There are two major types of binding. The covalent type of binding is irreversible and is, in general, associated with significant toxic effects. The noncovalent binding usually accounts for a major portion of the dose and is reversible. Therefore, this process plays an important role in the distribution of toxicants in various organs and tissues. There are several types of noncovalent binding as outlined by Guthrie (1980).

Plasma proteins can bind normal physiologic constituents in the body as well as some foreign compounds. Most of the latter are bound to the albumin and therefore not immediately available for distribution to the extravascular space. However, since the binding is reversible, it permits the bound chemical to dissociate from the protein, thereby replenishing the level of unbound chemical, which may then cross the capillary endothelium. The toxicologic significance of the binding can be illustrated by the possible induction of coma by the administration of sulfonamide drugs to patients who are taking antidiabetic drugs. The antidiabetic drugs are bound to the plasma proteins but can be replaced by the sulfonamide drugs, which have a greater affinity for the plasma protein. The antidiabetic drugs thus released may precipitate a hypoglycemic coma.

The *liver* and *kidney* have a higher capacity for binding chemicals. This characteristic may be related to their excretory and metabolic functions. Certain proteins have been identified in these organs for their specific binding property, e.g., metallothionein, which is important for the binding of cadmium in the liver and kidney and possibly also for the transfer of this metal from the liver to the kidney. Binding of a substance can increase its concentration in an organ rapidly. For example, 30 minutes after a single administration of lead, its concentration in the liver is 50 times higher than that in the plasma.

The *adipose tissue* is an important storage depot for lipid-soluble substances such as DDT, dieldrin, and polychlorinated biphenyls (PCB). They appear to be stored in the adipose tissue by simple dissolution in the neutral fats. There exists the potential that the plasma concentration of the substances stored in the fat may rise sharply as a result of rapid mobilization of fat following starvation. Conjugation of fatty acid to toxicants such as DDT may also be a mechanism by which these chemicals are retained in the lipid-containing tissues and cells of the body (Leighty et al., 1980).

Bone is a major site for storage for such toxicants as fluoride, lead, and strontium. The storage takes place by an exchange adsorption reaction between the toxicants in the interstitial fluid and the hydroxyapatite crystals of bone mineral. By virtue of similarities in size and charge, F^- may readily replace OH^-, and calcium may be replaced by lead or strontium. These stored substances can be released by ionic exchange and by dissolution of bone crystals through osteoclastic activity.

EXCRETION

After absorption and distribution in the organism, toxicants are excreted, rapidly or slowly. They are excreted as the parent chemicals, as their metabolites, and/or as conjugates of them. The principal route of excretion is the urine, but the liver and lungs are also important excretory organs for certain types of chemicals. In addition, there are a number of minor routes of excretion.

Urinary Excretion

The kidney removes toxicants from the body by the same mechanisms as those used in the removal of end-products of normal metabolism, namely, glomerular filtration, tubular diffusion, and tubular secretion.

The glomerular capillaries have large pores (40 Å); therefore, most toxicants will be filtered at the glomerulus, except those that are very large (greater than 60,000 mol. wt.) or are tightly bound to plasma protein. Once a toxicant enters the glomerular filtrate, it will either be passively reabsorbed across the tubular cells if it has a high lipid/water partition coefficient or remain in the tubular lumen and be excreted if it is a polar compound.

A toxicant can also be excreted through the tubules into the urine by passive diffusion. Since urine is normally acidic, this process plays a role in the excretion of organic bases. On the other hand, organic acids are unlikely to be excreted by passive diffusion through the tubular cells. However, weak acids are often metabolized to stronger acids, thereby increasing the percentage of the ionic forms that are not reabsorbed through the tubular cells and are thus excreted.

Certain toxicants can be secreted by the cells of the proximal tubules into the urine. There are two distinct secretory mechanisms, one for organic acids (e.g., glucuronide and sulfate conjugates) and the other for organic bases. Protein-bound toxicants can also be secreted, provided the binding is reversible. Furthermore, chemicals of similar characteristics compete for the same transport system. For example, probenecid can increase the serum level of penicillin and prolong its activity by blocking its tubular excretion.

Biliary Excretion

The liver is also an important organ for the excretion of toxicants, especially for compounds with high polarity (anionic and cationic), conjugates of compounds bound to plasma proteins, and compounds with molecular weights greater than 300. In general, once these compounds are in the bile, they are not reabsorbed into the blood and are excreted via the feces. However, there are exceptions, such as the glucuronide conjugates, which can be hydrolyzed by intestinal flora, enabling the reabsorption of the free toxicants.

The importance of the biliary route of excretion for some chemicals has been well demonstrated in experiments that showed a several fold increase of the acute toxicity in animals with ligated bile ducts. Such chemicals include digoxin, indocyanine green, ouabain, and, most dramatically, diethylstilbestrol (DES). The toxicity of DES is increased by a factor of 130 in rats with ligated bile ducts (Klaassen, 1973).

Lungs

Substances that exist in the gaseous phase at body temperature are excreted mainly by the lungs. Volatile liquids are also readily excreted via the expired air.

Highly soluble liquids such as chloroform and halothane may be excreted very slowly because of the limited ventilation volume as well as their storage in the adipose tissue. Excretion of toxicants from the lung is accomplished by simple diffusion through cell membranes.

Other Routes

The *gastrointestinal tract* is not a major route of excretion of toxicants. However, because the human stomach and intestine each secretes about 3 liters of fluid per day, some toxicants are excreted along with the fluid. The excretion is mainly by diffusion and thus the rate depends on the pK_a of the toxicant and the pH of the stomach and intestine.

The excretion of toxicants in mother's *milk* is not important as far as the host organism is concerned. However, the presence of toxic substances in milk is toxicologically significant because they can be passed in the milk from the mother to the nursing child and from cows to humans. The excretion is also via simple diffusion. Since milk is slightly acidic, basic compounds will reach a higher level in milk than in plasma, while the opposite is true with acidic compounds. Lipophilic compounds such as DDT and PCB also reach a higher level in milk because of its higher fat content.

Sweat and *saliva* are also minor routes of excretion of toxicants. The excretion is also by diffusion; thus it is confined to the nonionized, lipid-soluble forms of the toxicants. Substances excreted in the saliva are usually swallowed and then become available for absorption in the GI tract.

LEVELS OF TOXICANTS IN THE BODY

As noted above, the nature and intensity of the effects of a chemical depend on its concentration at the site of action, namely the effective dose rather than the administered dose. The level in the target organ is, in general, a function of the blood level. However, binding of a toxicant in a tissue will increase its level, whereas tissue barriers tend to reduce the level. Since the blood level is more readily determined, especially over a time period, it is the parameter often used in chemobiokinetic studies.

While the toxicant is being absorbed, its blood level rises. In the meantime, the rates of its excretion, biotransformation (see Chapter 3), and the distribution to other organs and tissues also increase. The curve depicting the blood level against time and the area under that curve (AUC) are useful tools in chemobiokinetics. In a series of experimental studies, Smyth and Hottendorf (1980) demonstrated that the AUC for a solution of a chemical is, in general, greater than that for its suspension, and it is greater for acidic than basic chemicals. They also illustrated the effects of the route of administration, dose level, and dosing vehicle on the AUC.

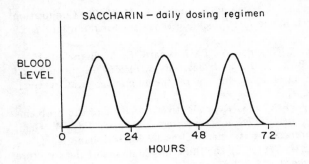

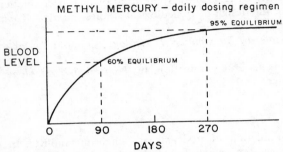

Figure 2-4 Comparative chemobiokinetics of saccharin and methyl mercury chloride (adapted from Munro and Willes, 1978, p. 138).

The influence of the rate of excretion on the blood level is vividly shown in Fig. 2-4. Saccharin is rapidly excreted; hence its blood level drops rapidly, even after repeated administration. On the other hand, methyl mercury is excreted very slowly; its gradual accumulation culminates in a near plateau only after 270 days (Munro and Willes, 1978).

REFERENCES

Bradbury, M. W. B. (1984) The structure and function of the blood-brain barrier. *Fed. Proc.* 43:186–190.

Guthrie, F. E. (1980) Absorption and distribution. In: *Introduction to Biochemical Toxicology*. Eds. E. Hodgson and F. E. Guthrie. New York: Elsevier.

Hatch, T., and Gross, P. (1964) *Pulmonary Deposition and Retention of Inhaled Aerosols*. New York: Academic Press.

Klaassen, C. D. (1973) Comparison of the toxicity of chemicals in newborn rats to bile duct-ligated and sham-operated rats and mice. *Toxicol. Apply. Pharmacol.* 24:37–44.

Leighty, E. G., Fentiman, A. F., Jr., and Thompson, R. M. (1980) Conjugation of fatty acids to DDT in the rat: Possible mechanism for retention. *Toxicology* 15:77–82.

Morrow, P. E., Hodge, H. C., Newman, W. F., Maynard, E. A., Blanchet, H. J., Jr., Fassett, D. W., Birk, R. E., and Mavrodt, S. (1966) Deposition and retention models for internal dosimetry of the human respiratory tract. *Health Phys.* 12:173–207.

Munro, I. O., and Willes, A. F. (1978) Reproductive toxicity and the problems of *in vitro* exposure. In: *Chemical Toxicology of Food.* Eds. A. Galli, R. Paoletti, and G. Veterazzi. Amsterdam: Elsevier/North Holland.

Singer, S. J., and Nicolson, G. C. (1972) The fluid mosaic model of the structure of cell membranes. *Science* 175:720–731.

Smyth, A. D., and Hottendorf, G. H. (1980) Application of pharmacokinetics and biopharmaceutics in the design of toxicological studies. *Toxicol. Appl. Pharmacol.* 53:179–195.

Timbrell, J. A. (1982) *Principles of Biochemical Toxicology.* London: Taylor & Francis.

Zbinden, G. (1976) Percutaneous drug permeation. In: *Progress in Toxicology*, Vol. 2. New York: Springer-Verlag.

ADDITIONAL READINGS

Matthews, H. B. (1980) Elimination of toxicants and their metabolites. In: *Introduction to Biochemical Toxicology.* Eds. E. Hodgson and F. E. Guthrie. New York: Elsevier.

WHO (1978) Principles and Methods for Evaluating the Toxicity of Chemicals. Part I. Environmental Health Criteria 6. Geneva: World Health Organization.

Chapter 3

Biotransformation
of Toxicants

GENERAL CONSIDERATIONS

As noted in the previous chapter, a toxicant can be absorbed into an organism via different routes. After absorption it is distributed to various parts of the body, including the excretory organs, and is thus available for excretion. Many chemicals are known to undergo biotransformation (metabolic transformation) while in the organs and tissues. The most important site of such reactions is the liver, the others being the lungs, stomach, intestine, skin, and kidneys.

Williams (1959) divided the biotransformation mechanisms into two major types:

1 Phase I reactions, involving oxidation, reduction, and hydrolysis
2 Phase II reactions, involving the production of a compound (a conjugate) that is biosynthesized from the toxicant, or its metabolite, plus an endogenous metabolite

Biotransformation is, therefore, a process that, in general, converts the parent compounds into metabolites and then forms conjugates. For example,

21

benzene undergoes oxidation, a phase I reaction, to form phenol, which conjugates with sulfate, a phase II reaction. However, when the administered chemical is phenol, it will conjugate with sulfate without a phase I reaction. The metabolites and conjugates are usually more water-soluble and more polar, hence more readily excretable. Biotransformation can therefore be considered a mechanism of detoxication by the host organism.

However, it must be noted that in certain cases the metabolites are more toxic than the parent compounds. Such reactions may be termed "bioactivation."

The rate of biotransformation and the type of biotransformation of a toxicant differ from one species of animal to another and even from one strain to another, a fact that often accounts for the difference of toxicity in these animals. The age and sex of the animal and exposures to other chemicals may also alter the biotransformation. Knowledge of such factors is important in the design of toxicologic studies and in the interpretation of health hazards of toxicants to humans.

DEGRADATION REACTIONS

The three types of phase I reactions, namely oxidation, reduction, and hydrolysis, will be briefly described, with examples taken from Hodgson and Dauterman (1980). A comprehensive summary of the reactions is given in Appendix 3-1.

Oxidation

The biotransformation of a great variety of chemicals involves oxidative processes. The most important enzyme systems catalyzing the processes involve cytochrome P-450 and NADPH cytochrome P-450 reductase. In these reactions, one atom of molecular oxygen is reduced to water and the other is incorporated into the substrate.

The cytochrome-linked mono-oxygenases (oxidases) are located in the endoplasmic reticulum. When a cell is homogenized, the endoplasmic reticulum breaks down to small vesicles known as microsomes. Because of the location of these enzymes and the great variety of chemicals that they may catalyze, they are also known as microsomal, mixed-function oxidases. In addition, oxidation of a number of toxicants is catalyzed by nonmicrosomal oxidoreductases that are located in the mitochrondrial fraction or in the 100,000-g supernatant of tissue homogenates.

Oxidation may take place in a variety of reactions, and often more than one metabolite is formed. The following are some examples:

A Microsomal oxidation

1 Aliphatic oxidation involves oxidation of the aliphatic side chains of aromatic chemicals: e.g., n-propylbenzene → 3-phenylpropan-1-ol, 3-phenyl-propan-2-ol, and 3-phenypropan-3-ol

2 Aromatic hydroxylation generally proceeds through an epoxide inter-mediate: e.g., naphthalene → naphthalene-1,2-epoxide → 1-naphthol + 2-naphthol

3 Epoxidation: e.g., aldrin → dieldrin

4 Oxidative deamination: e.g., amphetamine → phenylacetone

5 N-dealkylation: e.g., N,N-dimethyl-p-nitrophenyl carbamate → N-methyl-p-nitrophenyl carbamate

6 O-dealkylation: e.g., p-nitroanisole → p-nitrophenol

7 S-dealkylation: e.g., 6-methylthiopurine → 6-mercaptothiopurine

8 N-oxidation: e.g., trimethylamine → trimethylamine oxide

9 N-hydroxylation: e.g., aniline → phenylhydroxylamine

10 P-oxidation: e.g., diphenylmethylphosphine → diphenylmethylphos-phine oxide

11 Sulfoxidation: e.g., methiocarb → methiocarb sulfone

12 Desulfuration: e.g., parathion → paraoxon

B Nonmicrosomal oxidations

1 Amine oxidation: Monoamine oxidase is located in mitochondria and diamine oxidase is a soluble enzyme. Both are involved in the oxidation of the primary, secondary, and tertiary amines, such as 5-hydroxytryptamine and putrescine, into corresponding aldehydes.

2 Alcohol and aldehyde dehydrogenations are catalyzed, respectively, by alcohol dehydrogenase and aldehyde dehydrogenase: e.g., ethanol → acetalde-hyde → acetic acid

Reduction

Toxicants may undergo reductions through the function of reductases. These reactions are less active in mammalian tissues but more so in intestinal and intracellular bacteria. A notable example is the reduction of prontosil to sulfanil-amide.

A Microsomal reduction

1 Nitro reduction: e.g., nitrobenzene → nitrosobenzene → phenylhydroxyl-amine → aniline

2 Azo reduction: e.g., azobenzene → aniline

B Nonmicrosomal reductions occur via the reverse reaction of alcohol de-hydrogenases (see "Oxidation," B-2 above).

Hydrolysis

Many toxicants contain ester-type bonds and are subject to hydrolysis. These are essentially esters, amides, and compounds of phosphate. Mammalian tissues, including the plasma, contain a large number of nonspecific esterases and amidases, which are involved in hydrolysis. The esterases, usually located in the soluble fraction of the cell, may be broadly categorized into four classes (Testa and Jenner, 1976):

1 Arylesterases, which hydrolyze aromatic esters
2 Carboxylesterases, which hydrolyze aliphatic esters
3 Cholinesterases, which hydrolyze esters in which the alcohol moiety is choline
4 Acetylesterases, which hydrolyze esters in which the acid moiety is acetic acid

In contrast to esterases, amidases cannot be classified according to substrate specificity. Furthermore, enzymatic hydrolysis of amides proceeds much more slowly than that of esters, probably a result of the lack of substrate specificity.

CONJUGATION REACTIONS

Phase II reactions involve several types of endogenous metabolites that, as noted above, may form conjugates with the toxicants per se or their metabolites. These conjugates are generally more water-soluble and more readily excretable. Examples of each type of conjugation are also shown in Appendix 3-1.

Glucuronide Formation

This is the most common and most important type of conjugation. The enzyme catalyzing this reaction is UDP-glucuronyl transferase (uridine disphosphate glucuronyl transferase) and the coenzyme is UDPGA (uridine-5'-diphospho-α-D-glucuronic acid). This enzyme is also located in the endoplasmic reticulum. There are four classes of chemical compounds that are capable of forming conjugates with glucuronic acid: (1) aliphatic or aromatic alcohols, (2) carboxylic acids, (3) sulfhydryl compounds, and (4) amines.

Sulfate Conjugation

This reaction is catalyzed by sulfotransferases. These enzymes are found in the cytosolic fraction of liver, kidney, and interestine. The coenzyme is PAPS (3'-phosphoadenosine-5'-phosphosulfate). The functional groups of the foreign compounds for sulfate transfer are phenols and aliphatic alcohols as well as aromatic amines.

Methylation

This reaction is catalyzed by methyl transferases. The coenzyme is SAM (S-adenosylmethionine). Methylation is not a major route of biotransformation of toxicants because of the broader availability of UDPGA, which leads to the formation of glucuronides. Furthermore, it does not always increase the water solubility of the methylated products.

Acetylation

Acetylation involves transfer of acetyl groups to primary aromatic amines, hydrazines, hydrazides, sulfonamides, and certain primary aliphatic amines. The enzyme and coenzyme involved are respectively N-acetyl transferases and acetyl coenzyme A. In certain cases, acetylation results in a decrease in water solubility of an amine and an increase in toxicity (see "Bioactivation").

Amino Acid Conjugation

This conjugation is catalyzed by amino acid conjugates and coenzyme A. Aromatic carboxylic acids, arylacetic acids, aryl-substituted acrylic acids can form conjugates with α-amino acids, mainly glycine, but also glutamine in humans and certain monkeys and ornithine in birds.

Glutathione Conjugation

This important reaction is effected by glutathione S-transferases and the cofactor glutathione. Glutathione conjugates subsequently undergo enzymatic cleavage and acetylation, forming N-acetylcysteine (mercapturic acid) derivatives of the toxicants, which are readily excreted. Examples of chemicals such as epoxides and aromatic halogens that conjugate with glutathione are shown in Fig. 3-1. In addition, glutathione can conjugate unsaturated aliphatic compounds and displace nitro groups in chemicals.

In the process of biotransformation of toxicants, a number of highly reactive electrophilic compounds are formed. Some of these compounds can react with cellular constituents and cause cell death or induce tumor formation. The role of glutathione is to react with the electrophilic compounds and thus prevent their harmful effects on the cells. However, exposure to very large amounts of such reactive substances can deplete the glutathione, thereby resulting in marked toxic effects. An example of the depletion of glutathione by acetaminophen and the concomitant increase in covalent binding to macromolecules is shown in Fig. 3-2.

BIOACTIVATION

Certain chemically stable compounds can be converted to chemically reactive metabolites. These reactive compounds can become covalently bound to tissue

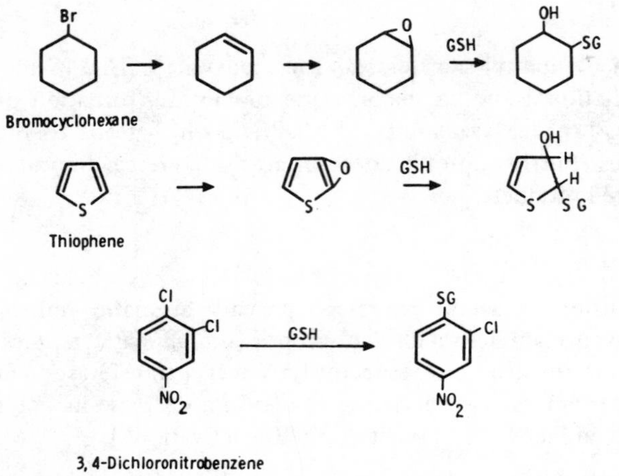

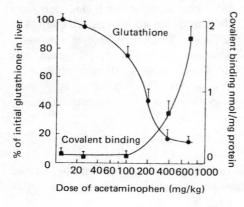

Bromocyclohexane

Thiophene

3, 4-Dichloronitrobenzene

Figure 3-1 Conjugation of epoxide and dehalogenation catalyzed by glutathione (GSH) transferase (from Timbrell, 1982).

macromolecules and cause injury. In addition, other types of metabolites produce toxic effects via other mechanisms.

Appendix 3-2 lists a variety of bioactivations.

Epoxide Formation

Many aromatic compounds are converted to epoxides by microsomal mixed-function oxygenase systems. The biotransformation of bromobenzene to its epoxide and subsequent reactions serve as an interesting example of bioactivation and its consequences. These are depicted in Fig. 3-3.

Although bromobenzene epoxide may become covalently bound to tissue macromolecules and cause injury, the alternative routes of metabolism may prevent or reduce the injury. The most important of these routes is the conjugation

Figure 3-2 Protective effect of glutathione against covalent binding of acetaminophen to liver proteins (from Wills, 1981).

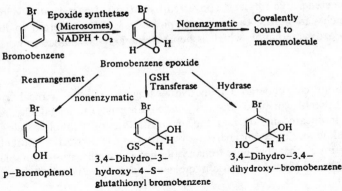

Figure 3-3 The bromobenzene epoxide formed from the parent chemical may covalently bind to macromolecules, but such binding may be minimal when the other metabolic routes are predominant (from Gillette and Mitchell, 1975).

with glutathione (catalyzed by GSH transferase). This reaction is important in that it serves as a protective mechanism. Only after the hepatic levels of reduced glutathione have been greatly depleted will the bromobenzene epoxide significantly bind to macromolecules and result in hepatic necrosis. Depletion of glutathione occurs when a huge dose of bromobenzene is present or when there has been an induction of microsomal enzymes; both conditions increase the amount of bromobenzene epoxide. Other reactions include a nonenzymatic arrangement to form p-bromophenol and the formation of 3,4-dihydro-3,4-dihydroxy-bromobenzene catalyzed by hydrase.

As listed in Appendix 3-2, the epoxide metabolites are probably the ultimate carcinogens of such chemicals as aflatoxin B_1 and polycyclic hydrocarbons.

N-Hydroxylation

Microsomal enzymes from many tissues can N-hydroxylate a variety of chemicals. Some of the N-hydroxy metabolites, such as those of certain aminoazo dyes and acetaminophen, can cause cancer or tissue necrosis through covalent binding, whereas others, e.g., certain aromatic amines, can induce hemolysis or methemoglobinemia (Appendix 3-2).

N-Hydroxy metabolites are also subject to conjugation reactions. Their conjugates with glucuronic acid are readily excreted; those formed with sulfuric or acetic acid, however, may be unstable and thus can be mutagenic, carcinogenic, and highly toxic (Weisburger and Weisburger, 1973).

Activation in the GI Tract

Nitrites and certain amines can react in the acidic environment of the stomach to form nitrosamines, many of which have been shown to be potent carcinogens.

The artificial sweetener cyclamate is converted by intestinal bacteria to cyclo-hexylamine, which can induce testicular atrophy. Cycasin is converted to its aglycone, methylazoxymethanol, which is hepatotoxic and can induce tumors.

Other Pathways

Carbon tetrachloride can undergo a reductive cleavage to the free radical tri-chloromethane. Ethanol can be oxidized by a dehydrogenase to acetaldehyde, which has been implicated in some of the manifestations of alcohol toxicity. Pyrrolizidine alkaloids are dehydrogenated to reactive pyrrole derivatives. Recent evidence has confirmed that the acute toxicity of aliphatic nitriles is attributable to the cyanide released through hepatic microsomal enzyme activities (Willhite and Smith, 1981).

COMPLEX NATURE OF BIOTRANSFORMATION

Toxicants generally undergo several types of biotransformation, resulting in a variety of metabolites and conjugates. Some of the various metabolites and conjugates of bromobenzene are shown in Fig. 3-3, and those of carbaryl are shown in Fig. 3-4. Organophosphorous insecticides, such as fenithrothion, chlorofenvinphos, omethoate, can be metabolized through dealkylation, oxida-tion, desulfuration, or hydrolysis, yielding ten or more different metabolites (WHO, 1969; 1971).

Parathion, an organophosphorous pesticide, is bioactivated in the liver to paraoxon, which is a much more potent cholinesterase inhibitor. Infusion of parathion by way of the vena cava, bypassing the liver, therefore, produced little cholinesterase inhibition, but a moderate effect was induced following infusion by way of the portal vein. On the other hand, infusion of paraoxon via the vena cava nearly completely blocked the cholinesterase activity, whereas it had negligible effect after an infusion via the portal vein, since it is detoxicated in the liver (Westermann, 1961).

The relative importance of various types of biotransformation of a toxicant depends on many host, environmental, and chemical factors as well as the dose of the toxicant. Since the metabolites resulting from different biotransforma-tions are often markedly different in their effects, the toxicity of a chemical can be greatly altered by these factors, as will be discussed in Chapter 5.

Some of the metabolic reactions take place in sequence; hence interference of the normal metabolic pathway may have considerable influence on the toxic effects. For example, ethanol is normally metabolized through the intermediary product acetaldehyde. In normal humans the acetaldehyde formed is rapidly further metabolized to acetate, which in turn is converted to carbon dioxide and water. However, if the aldehyde dehydrogenase is inhibited, such as after the administration of disulfiram, the level of acetaldehyde rises and results in distress symptoms such as nausea, vomiting, headache, and palpitations.

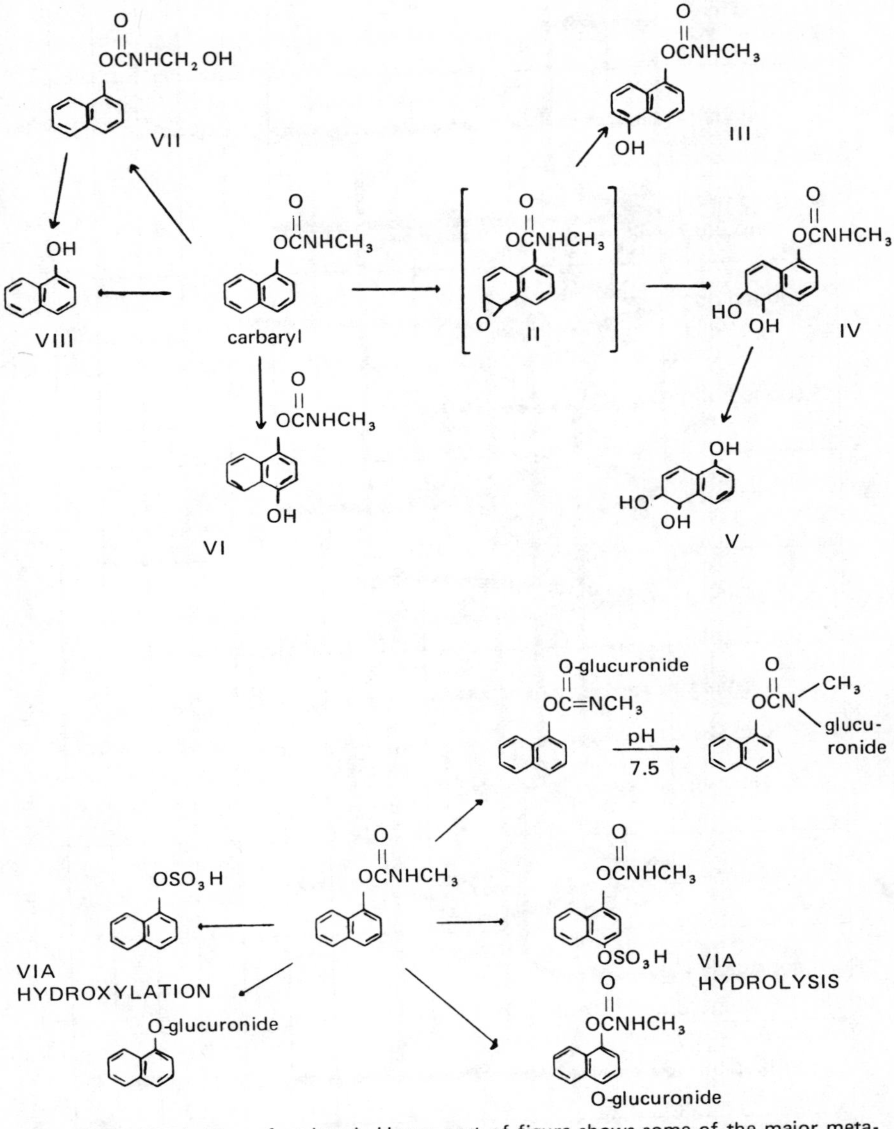

Figure 3-4 Metabolites of carbaryl. Upper part of figure shows some of the major metabolites found in in vitro studies using mammalian liver microsomes; lower part shows the major metabolites found in the urine of mammals (from Fukuto and Metcalf, 1969).

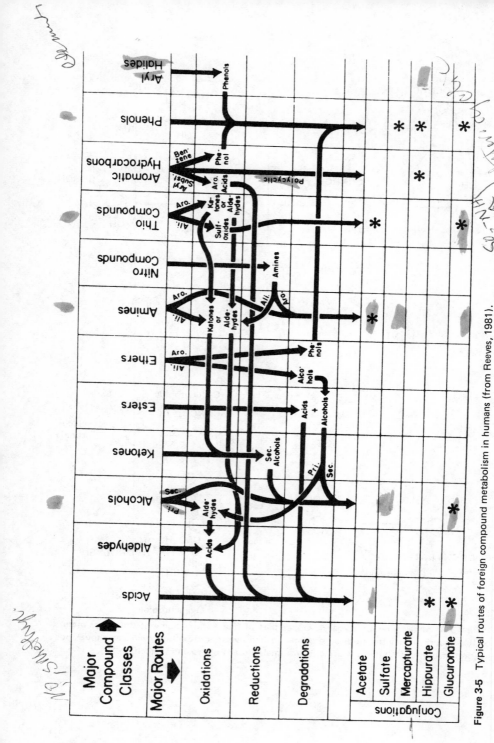

Figure 3-5 Typical routes of foreign compound metabolism in humans (from Reeves, 1981).

A somewhat similar situation exists with methanol. It is metabolized to formaldehyde and then to formate, which in turn converts to carbon dioxide and water. However, the human eye lacks the specific enzyme to oxidize formaldehyde to formate. Hence, human exposure to methanol will result in an accumulation of formaldehyde in the eye. As this chemical is locally destructive, repeated exposure can lead to total blindness.

Reeves (1981) provides a number of examples of biotransformations of "typical" chemicals, as well as a limited generalization of the typical routes of foreign compound metabolism in humans (Fig. 3-5).

APPENDIXES

Appendix 3-1   Metabolic Transformations

I. OXIDATIONS

(a) *Microsomal oxidations*

Aliphatic oxidation

$$RCH_3 \longrightarrow RCH_2OH$$

Aromatic hydroxylation

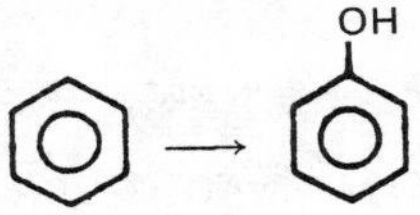

Epoxidation

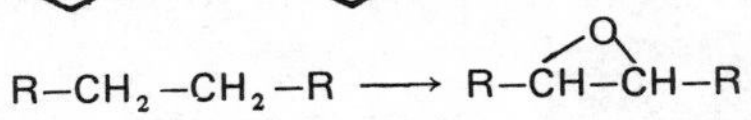

$$R-CH_2-CH_2-R \longrightarrow R-\overset{\displaystyle O}{\overset{\diagup\ \diagdown}{CH-CH}}-R$$

Oxidative deamination

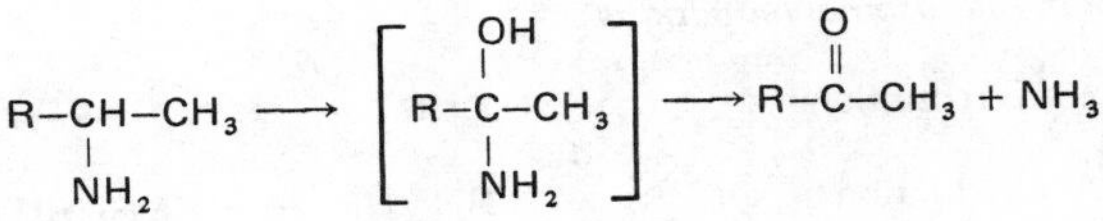

$$R-\underset{\underset{NH_2}{|}}{CH}-CH_3 \longrightarrow \left[R-\underset{\underset{NH_2}{|}}{\overset{\overset{OH}{|}}{C}}-CH_3 \right] \longrightarrow R-\overset{\overset{O}{\|}}{C}-CH_3 + NH_3$$

N-dealkylation

$$R-N\overset{\diagup CH_3}{\diagdown CH_3} \longrightarrow R-N\overset{\diagup H}{\diagdown CH_3} + CH_2O$$

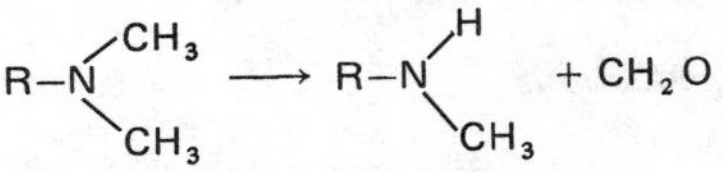

O-dealkylation

$$R-O-CH_3 \longrightarrow R-OH + CH_2O$$

S-dealkylation

$$R-S-CH_3 \longrightarrow R-SH + CH_2O$$

Metaloalkane dealkylation

$$Pb(C_2H_5)_4 \longrightarrow PbH(C_2H_5)_3$$

N-oxidation

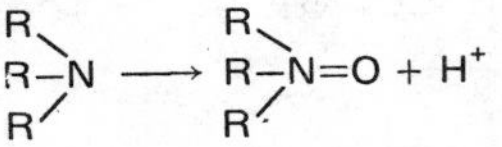

$$\overset{\overset{\displaystyle R}{\diagdown}}{\underset{\underset{\displaystyle R}{\diagup}}{R-N}} \longrightarrow \overset{\overset{\displaystyle R}{\diagdown}}{\underset{\underset{\displaystyle R}{\diagup}}{R-N}}=O + H^+$$

Source: WHO (1978)

Appendix 3-1   Metabolic Transformations (*Continued*)

N-hydroxylation	NH$_2$ → NHOH

Sulfoxidation	R–S–R → R–$\overset{O}{\underset{\uparrow}{S}}$–R

Desulfuration	$\overset{R}{\underset{R}{>}}$C=S → $\overset{R}{\underset{R}{>}}$C=O

Dehalogenation	F → OH

(b) Nonmicrosomal oxidations

Monoamine and diamine oxidation	$RCH_2NH_2 \xrightarrow{O_2} RCH=NH \xrightarrow{H_2O} RCHO + NH_3$
Alcohol dehydrogenation	$RCH_2OH + NAD^+ \longrightarrow R-CHO + NADH + H^+$
Aldehyde dehydrogenation	$R-CHO + NAD^+ \longrightarrow R-COOH + NADH + H^+$

II. REDUCTIONS

(a) Microsomal reductions

Nitro reduction	$RNO_2 \longrightarrow RNO \longrightarrow RNHOH \longrightarrow RNH_2$
Azo reduction	$RN=NR \longrightarrow RNHNHR \longrightarrow RNH_2 + RNH_2$
Reductive dehalogenation	$R-CCl_3 \longrightarrow R-CHCl_2$

(b) Nonmicrosomal reductions

Aldehyde reduction	$\overset{R}{\underset{R}{>}}$C=O → $\overset{R}{\underset{R}{>}}$CHOH

III. HYDROLYSIS

Ester hydrolysis	$R-CO-O-R_1 \longrightarrow R-COOH + R_1-OH$
Amide hydrolysis	$R-CO-NH_2 \longrightarrow R-COOH + NH_3$

Appendix 3-1 Metabolic Transformations (*Continued*)

IV. CONJUGATION

(a) *UDPGA-mediated conjugations*

O-glucuronide formation
ether type:

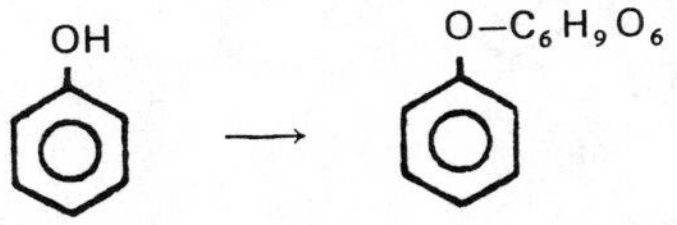

$OH \longrightarrow O-C_6H_9O_6$

ester type:

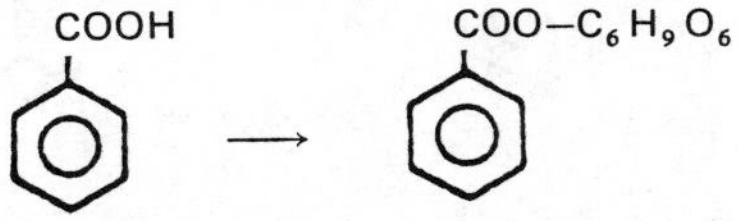

$COOH \longrightarrow COO-C_6H_9O_6$

N-glucuronide formation

$NH_2 \longrightarrow NH-C_6H_9O_6$

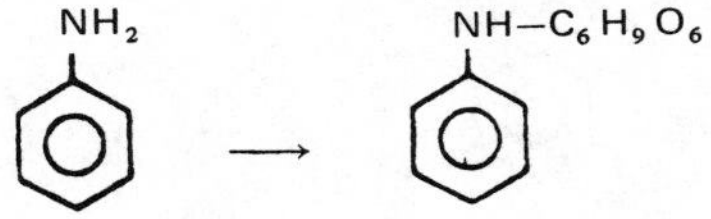

S-glucuronide formation

$SH \longrightarrow S-C_6H_9O_6$

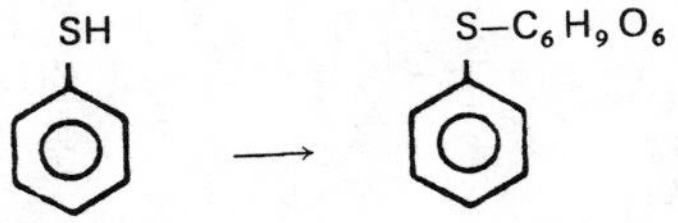

(b) *PAPS-mediated conjugation*

Sulfate ester formation

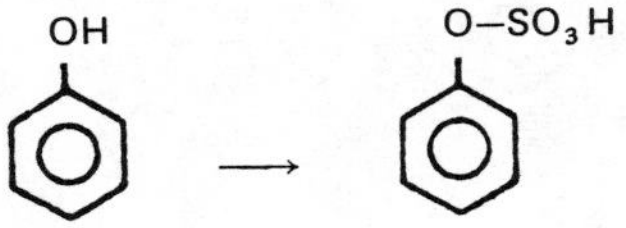

$OH \longrightarrow O-SO_3H$

$C_2H_5OH \longrightarrow C_2H_5O-SO_3H$

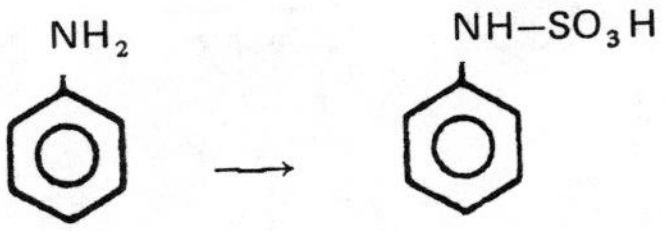

$NH_2 \longrightarrow NH-SO_3H$

Appendix 3-1 Metabolic Transformations (*Continued*)

(*c*) *Methylations*

N-methylation

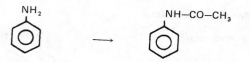

O-methylation

S-methylation $C_2H_5SH \longrightarrow C_2H_5S-CH_3$

(*d*) *Acetylations*

(*e*) *Peptide conjugations*

$\dfrac{ATP,CoA}{glycine}$

(*f*) *Glutathione conjugations*

GSH

Appendix 3-2   Examples of Bioactivation

Parent compound	Toxic metabolite	Site of formation	Mechanism of toxicity	Toxicity	References
Acetaminophen	N-Hydroxy derivative	Liver	Covalent binding	Hepatic necrosis	Mitchell et al. (1973a), Jollow et al. (1973), Potter et al. (1973), Mitchell et al. (1973b)
2-Acetylaminofluorene (AAF)	N-Acetoxy-AAF, AAF N-sulfate	Liver	Covalent binding	Cancers	Weisburger and Weisburger (1973)
Aflatoxin B₁	Aflatoxin-2,3-epoxide?	Liver	Covalent binding	Hepatic cancer	Lijinsky et al. (1970), Garner et al. (1972), Swenson et al. (1973)
Allyl-containing barbiturates	Epoxide?	Liver	Unknown	Hepatic cytochrome P-450 destruction, porphyria	Foreman and Maynert (1970), Levin et al. (1973)
Allyl formate	Acrolein	Liver	Covalent binding?	Hepatic necrosis	Rees and Tarlow (1967)
Allylisopropylacetamide	Epoxide?	Liver	Unknown	Hepatic cytochrome P-450 destruction, porphyria	Doedens (1971), De Matteis (1973a)
Amygdalin	Mandelonitrile	Gut flora	Cyanide formation	Cytotoxic hypoxia	Williams (1972)
Benzene	Benzene epoxide	Liver	Covalent binding	Bone marrow depression	Jerina et al. (1968), Mitchell (1971), Gonasun et al. (1973)
Bromobenzene	Bromobenzene epoxide	Liver, lung	Covalent binding	Hepatic, renal bronchiolar necrosis	Reid (1973b), Reid and Krishna (1973), Reid et al. (1973)
Carbon tetrachloride	Trichloromethane free radical	Liver	Covalent binding	Hepatic necrosis, hepatic cancer	Slater (1966), Uehleke et al. (1973), Krishna et al. (1973)

Source: Mazel and Pessayre, 1976.

Appendix 3-2 Examples of Bioactivation (*Continued*)

Parent compound	Toxic metabolite	Site of formation	Mechanism of toxicity	Toxicity	References
Carcinogenic alkylnitrosamines	Unknown	Liver, many organs?	Alkylation	Hepatic cancer	Magee and Barnes (1967), Magee et al. (1973)
Carcinogenic aminoazo dyes	N-Hydroxy derivatives	Liver	Covalent binding	Hepatic cancer	Poirier and Weisburger (1973)
Carcinogenic polycyclic hydrocarbons	Epoxides?	Many organs	Covalent binding	Cancers cytotoxicity	Boyland (1950, 1964), Grover et al. (1971), Philips et al. (1973), Magee (1974)
Chloramphenicol	Unknown	Liver, bone marrow	Covalent binding	Aplasia	Krishna and Bonanomi (1974)
Chloroform	Unknown	Liver, kidney?	Covalent binding	Hepatic, renal necrosis	Illett et al. (1973)
Cycasin	Methylazoxy-methanol	Gut flora	Alkylation	Cancers, hepatic necrosis	Laqueur (1968)
Cyclamate	Cyclohexylamine	Gut flora	Unknown	Bladder cancer	Price et al. (1970), Drasar et al. (1972), Renwick and Williams (1972)
Cyclophosphamide	Many proposed	Liver, lung	Alkylation	Cytotoxic	Hayes et al. (1972), Short and Gibson (1974), Torkelson et al. (1974)
Ethanol	Acetaldehyde	Many organs	Complex	Varied	Beck et al. (1968), Cohen and Collins (1970), Truitt and Walsh (1971), Raskin and Sokoloff (1972)
Fluoroacetate	Fluorocitrate	Many organs	Enzyme inhibition	General toxicity	Peters (1955, 1957)
Furosemide	Epoxide?	Liver	Covalent binding	Hepatic, renal necrosis	Mitchell et al. (1974a)
Halothane	Unknown	Liver	Covalent binding?	Hepatic necrosis	Van Dyke and Wood (1973), Reynolds and Moslen (1974), Hempel and Remmer (1975)

Compound	Active metabolite	Organ	Mechanism	Toxic effect	Reference
Hemolysis-producing aromatic amines	N-Hydroxy metabolites	Liver	Unknown	Hemolysis	Mitchell and Jollow (1974)
Isoniazid	Acetylhydrazine (metabolite of)	Liver	Covalent binding	Hepatic necrosis	Mitchell and Jollow (1974)
Meclizine	Norchlorcyclizine?	Liver?	Unknown	Teratogenesis	King (1963), King et al. (1965), Narrod et al. (1965)
Methanol	Formaldehyde	Liver, retina	Complex	Retinal and general toxicity	Cooper and Kini (1962), Kini and Cooper (1962)
Methemoglobin-producing aromatic amines and nitro compounds	N-Hydroxy metabolites	Liver, other organs	Cyclic oxido-reduction	Methemoglobinemia	Uehleke (1973b)
Methoxyflurane	Inorganic fluoride	Liver	Enzyme inhibition?	Renal failure	Mazze and Cousins (1973)
Mitotane (o,p'-DDD)	Unknown	Adrenal	Covalent binding	Adrenal necrosis	Martz and Straw (1975)
Naphthylamine	N-Hydroxy naphthylamine?	Liver	Covalent binding	Bladder cancer	Boyland (1958), Radomski and Brill (1970)
Nitrates	Nitrites	Gut flora	Hemoglobin oxidation	Methemoglobin	Nason (1962), Wolff and Wasserman (1972)
Nitrites plus secondary or tertiary amines	Nitrosamines	Stomach	Alkylation	Hepatic, pulmonary cancers	Lijinsky et al. (1972a), Lijinsky et al. (1972b), Lijinsky et al. (1973)
Nitrofurazone	Unknown	Liver, testis	Covalent binding	Mammary tumors, testicular degeneration	Stripp et al. (1973a)
Olefins	Epoxides	Liver	Covalent binding?	Skin cancer	Van Duuren et al. (1967), Leibman and Ortiz (1970), Watabe and Akamatsu (1974), Watabe and Yamada (1975)

Appendix 3-2 Examples of Bioactivation (*Continued*)

Parent compound	Toxic metabolite	Site of formation	Mechanism of toxicity	Toxicity	References
Parathion	Paraoxon	Liver	Covalent binding to cholinesterase	Neuromuscular paralysis	Davies and Green (1958), Hitchcock and Murphy (1971)
Phalloidin and α-amanitin	Unknown	Liver?	Unknown	Hepatic, renal necrosis	Floersheim (1966a, 1966b)
Purine and pyrimidine base analogues	Mononucleotides, nucleotide triphosphates	Diffuse	Lethal synthesis, lethal incorporation	Cytotoxicity	Mandel (1959)
Pyrrolizidine alkaloids	Pyrrolic derivatives	Liver	Unknown	Hepatic necrosis, lung edema	Jago et al. (1970), Mattocks and White (1971), Mattocks (1972), White et al. (1973)
Safrole	1'-Hydroxysafrole (metabolite of)	Unknown	Covalent binding	Cancers	Borchert et al. (1973a), Borchert et al. (1973b)
Spironolactone	Unknown	Testis, adrenal	Unknown	Testicular or adrenal cytochrome P-450 destruction	Stripp et al. (1973b), Menard and Stripp (1974), Menard et al. (1974)
Thalidomide	Phthalyl-L-glutamic acid?	Nonenzymatic hydrolysis	Unknown	Teratogenesis	Williams (1963), Keberle et al. (1965), Ockenfels and Kohler (1970)
Urethane	N-Hydroxy-urethane	Liver	Alkylation	Cancers, cytotoxicity	Boyland and Nery (1965)

REFERENCES

Fukuto, T. R., and Metcalf, R. L. (1969) Metabolism of insecticides in plants and animals. *Ann. NY Acad. Sci.* 160:97–113.

Gillette, J. R., and Mitchell, J. R. (1975) Drug actions and interactions: Theoretical considerations. In: *Handbook of Experimental Pharmacology. New Series*, Vol. 28, pp. 359–382. Eds. O. Eichler, A. Farah, H. Herken, and A. D. Welch. New York: Springer-Verlag.

Hodgson, E., and Dauterman, W. C. (1980) Metabolism of toxicants: Phase I reactions. In: *Introduction to Biochemical Toxicology*. Eds. E. Hodgson and F. E. Guthrie. New York: Elsevier.

Mazel, P., and Pessayre, D. (1976) Significance of metabolite-mediated toxicities in the safety evaluation of drugs and chemicals. In: *New Concept in Safety Evaluation. Vol. 1, Part 1*. Eds. M. A. Mehlmen, R. E. Shapiro, and H. Blumenthal. Washington, D.C.: Hemisphere.

Reeves, A. L. (1981) The metabolism of foreign compounds. In: *Toxicology: Principles and Practices, Vol. 1*. Ed. Reeves. New York: John Wiley.

Testa, B., and Jenner, P. (1976) *Drug Metabolism: Chemical and Biochemical Aspects*. New York: Marcel Dekker.

Timbrell, J. A. (1982) *Principles of Biochemical Toxicology*. London: Taylor & Francis.

Weisburger, J. H., and Weisburger, E. K. (1973) Biochemical formation and pharmacological, toxicological and pathological properties of hydroxylamines and hydroxamic acids. *Pharmacol. Rev.* 25:1–66.

Westerman, E. O. (1961) *Introduction to General Toxicology*, p. 147. Eds. E. J. Ariens, A. M. Simonis, and J. Offermeier, 1976. New York: Academic Press.

WHO (1969) Fenithrothion. In: *1969 Evaluation of Pesticide Residue in Foods*. Geneva: World Health Organization.

WHO (1971) Chlorfenvinphos and Omethoate. In: *1972 Evaluations of Some Pesticide Residues in Food*. Geneva: World Health Organization.

WHO (1978) Metabolic transformation. In: *Environmental Health Criteria 6*. Geneva: World Health Organization.

Willhite, C. C., and Smith, R. P. (1981) The role of cyanide liberation in the acute toxicity of aliphatic nitriles. *Toxicol. Appl. Pharmacol.* 59:589–602.

Williams, R. T. (1959) *Detoxication Mechanisms*, 2d ed. London: Chapman & Hall.

Wills, E. D. (1981) The role of glutathione in drug metabolism and the protection of the liver against toxic metabolites. In: *Testing for Toxicity*. Ed. J. W. Gorrod. London: Taylor & Francis.

ADDITIONAL READINGS

Dauterman, W. C. (1980) Metabolism of toxicants: Phase II reactions. In: *Introduction to Biochemical Toxicology*. Eds. E. Hodgson and F. E. Guthrie. New York: Elsevier.

Neal, R. A. (1980) Metabolism of toxic substances. In: *Casarett and Doull's Toxicology*. Eds. J. Doull, C. D. Klaassen, and M. O. Amdur. New York: Macmillan.

Chapter 4

Toxic Effects

GENERAL CONSIDERATIONS

Toxic effects are greatly variable in nature, target organ, and mechanism of action. A better understanding of their characteristics can improve assessment of the associated health hazards. It can also facilitate the development of rational preventive and therapeutic measures.

All toxic effects result from biochemical interactions between the toxicants (and/or their metabolites) and certain structures of the organism. The structure may be nonspecific, such as any tissue in direct contact with corrosive chemicals. More often it is specific, involving a particular subcellular structure. A variety of structures, including the "receptors," may be affected.

The nature of effects may vary from organ to organ. The organ-specific effects will be discussed in some detail in the chapters in Part III. In some cases, the reason why a particular organ is affected is known. This knowledge is useful in many ways. A few examples are described in this chapter.

40

CATEGORIES OF TOXIC EFFECTS

The great variety of toxic effects can be grouped in different ways, some of which are discussed below:

Local and Systemic Effects

Certain chemicals can cause injuries at the site of first contact with an organism. These local effects can be induced by caustic substances on the gastrointestinal tract, by corrosive materials on the skin, and by irritant gases and vapors on the respiratory tract. Such local effects represent generalized destruction of living cells.

Systemic effects result only after the toxicant has been absorbed and distributed to other parts of the body. Most toxicants exert their main effects on one or a few organs. These organs are referred to as the "target organs" of these toxicants. A target organ does not necessarily have the highest concentration of the toxicants in the organism. For example, the target organ of methyl mercury is the central nervous system, but its concentration is much higher in the liver and kidney. Likewise, the target organ of DDT is also the central nervous system, but it is concentrated in adipose tissues.

Reversible and Irreversible Effects

Reversible effects of toxicants are those that will disappear following cessation of exposure to them. Irreversible effect, in contrast, will persist or even progress after exposure is discontinued. Certain effects are obviously irreversible. These include carcinomas, mutations, damages to the neurons, and liver cirrhosis.

Certain effects are considered irreversible even though they disappear some time after cessation of exposure. For example, the "irreversible" cholinesterase-inhibiting insecticides inhibit the activity of this enzyme for a period of time that approximates that required for the synthesis and replacement of the enzyme.

The effect produced by a toxicant may be reversible if the organism is exposed at a low concentration and/or for a short duration, whereas irreversible effects may be produced at higher concentrations and/or for longer durations of exposure.

Immediate and Delayed Effects

Many toxicants produce immediate toxic effects, which develop shortly after a single exposure, a notable example being cyanide poisoning. Delayed effects occur after a lapse of some time. Carcinogenic effects generally become manifest 10–20 years after the initial exposure in humans; even in rodents a lapse of many months is required. To determine these and other delayed effects of toxicants, long-term studies are essential.

Morphologic, Functional, and Biochemical Effects

Morphologic effects refer to gross and microscopic changes in the morphology of the tissues. Many of these effects, e.g., necrosis, neoplasia, are irreversible and serious. Functional effects usually represent reversible changes in the functions of target organs. Functions of the liver and kidney (e.g., rate of excretion of dyes) are commonly tested in toxicologic studies.

Since functional effects are in general reversible, whereas morphologic effects are not, several investigations have attempted to show that functional changes might be detected earlier or in animals exposed to lower doses than those with morphologic changes. The evidence collected in certain hepatic and renal tests, however, does not support this assumption (Sharratt and Frazer, 1963; Grice, 1972; Zbinden, 1976). However, more recent findings indicate that certain functional tests are more sensitive. In addition, functional tests are valuable in following the progress of effects on target organs in long-term studies in animals and in humans.

Although all toxic effects are associated with biochemical alterations, in routine toxicity testing, "biochemical effects" usually refer to those without apparent morphologic changes. An example of such effects is the elevation of serum transaminases, which is associated usually with toxic effects on the liver but occasionally with myocardial infarction and muscle injury. Some biochemical effects represent changes in functions. These include the toxic manifestations associated with cholinesterase inhibition following exposure to organophosphate and carbamate insecticides.

Allergic and Idiosyncratic Reactions

Allergic reaction to a toxicant results from previous sensitization to that toxicant or a chemically similar one. The chemical acts as a hapten and combines with an endogenous protein to form an antigen, which in turn elicits the formation of antibodies. A subsequent exposure to the chemical will result in an antigen-antibody interaction, which provokes the typical manifestations of allergy. Thus this reaction is different from the usual toxic effects, first because a previous exposure is required, and second because a typical sigmoid dose-response curve is usually not demonstrable with allergic reactions (Loomis, 1978). Nevertheless, threshold doses were demonstrable for the induction as well as the challenge in dermal sensitization (Koschier et al., 1983).

Generally an idiosyncratic reaction is a genetically determined abnormal reactivity to a chemical. Some patients exhibit prolonged muscular reaction and apnea following a standard dose of succinylcholine. These patients have a deficiency of serum cholinesterase, which normally degrades the muscle relaxant rapidly. Similarly, people with a deficiency in NADH methemoglobinemia reductase are abnormally sensitive to nitrites and other chemicals that produce methemoglobinemia.

TARGET ORGANS

Toxicants do not affect all organs to the same extent. The reason is not always clear. For example, methoxyflurane is metabolized to release F^-. This takes place in the liver, but the toxicity is exerted on the kidney. Presumably, for some reason, the kidney is more sensitive than the liver (Mazze and Cousins, 1973). On the other hand, the probable mechanisms by which toxicants act specifically on certain organs are as follows.

Distribution

Being lipophilic, methyl mercury can cross the blood-brain barrier and exert its toxic effects on the nervous system. Inorganic mercury compounds, in contrast, are not able to cross the blood-brain barrier and are not neurotoxic.

Many toxicants exert their effects on the liver and kidney because of the high concentrations in these excretory organs.

The respiratory tract and the skin are target organs of certain industrial and environmental toxicants because these are the sites of absorption.

Sensitivity of the Organ

Neurons and myocardium depend primarily on adenosine triphosphate (ATP) generated by mitochondrial oxidation with little capacity for anaerobic metabolism and there are rapid ionic shifts through the cell membrane. They are, therefore, especially sensitive to lack of oxygen resulting from disorders of the vascular system or of the hemoglobin (e.g., carbon monoxide poisoning).

Rapidly dividing cells, such as those in the bone marrow and those in the intestinal mucosa, are more susceptible to mitotic poisons.

Biotransformation

Methanol is normally metabolized through formaldehyde and formate to carbon dioxide and water. The human eye, however, lacks the enzyme to metabolize formaldehyde to formate and, therefore is especially susceptible to the toxicity of methanol.

The liver is an important site of bioactivation of many toxicants; hence liver is a common target organ. However, if the metabolites are sufficiently stable, they may affect other organs after being transported there (e.g., bromobenzene on the kidney).

Other Factors

The phosphorothioate insecticides are mainly bioactivated in the liver, but the abundance of detoxifying enzymes and of reactive but noncritical binding sites there prevent any overt signs of toxicity. On the other hand, brain tissue has much less of such bioactivating enzymes, but because the bioactivation takes place near the critical target sites, i.e., the synapses, the main toxic manifestations of this group of toxicants arise from the central nervous system. References to the above and several other examples are cited in a WHO document (1978).

A toxicant may affect a specific organ because of a lack of the required repair mechanism. For example, N-methyl-N-nitrosourea (MNU) produces tumors in the rat mainly in the brain, occasionally in the kidney, but never in the liver. Kleihues and Cooper (1976) demonstrated that the liver is fully capable of enzymatically excising the O^6-alkyl-guanine induced by MNU from the DNA, whereas the brain is deficient in this respect. The capacity of the kidney falls between those of the liver and brain.

MECHANISM OF ACTION

The mechanism of action underlying an overt toxic effect can usually be defined by changes at one or more subcellular sites. The potential sites are the nuclei, mitochondria, lysosomes, endoplasmic reticulum, other cell bodies, and plasma membranes. The mechanism can also be classified by the chemical nature of the molecular targets. These include proteins, coenzymes, lipids, and nucleic acids. Carbohydrates, on the other hand, are rarely affected by toxicants.

Proteins

Structural Proteins Structural proteins such as plasma and organelle membranes are more commonly damaged. Notable examples are hexane and silica. Such damages result in impairment of the structural as well as other functions of the membranes. On the other hand, the structural protein collagen is rarely affected.

Enzymes Enzymes are common targets of toxicants. The enzyme effects may be specific, such as the inhibition of acetylcholinesterase. They may be reversible, such as the case with a number of carbamate insecticides on cholinesterase. Irreversible enzyme inhibition is exemplified by DFP (diisopropyl fluorophosphate) and monoamine oxidase inhibitors, which covalently bind with the enzymes.

The effects may be nonspecific. For example, lead and mercury are inhibitors of a great variety of enzymes. However, some enzymes are more susceptible, e.g., aminolevulinic acid dehydrase is especially sensitive to lead and its activity in erythrocytes is used as an early indicator of lead poisoning.

The last step of the oxidation of many chemicals is catalyzed by the cytochrome oxidase chain. Hydrocyanic acid (HCN) can bind with the iron in these enzymes and block their redox function. The aerobic respiration of cells is then arrested and biochemical asphyxia ensues.

An enzyme can also be inhibited by a chemical derived by synthesis from the toxicant such as fluoroacetic acid and its derivatives. The process is known as lethal synthesis. Fluoroacetic acid is metabolized as acetic acid in the citric cycle, and fluorocitric acid is synthesized, instead of citric acid. Since fluorocitric acid is an inhibitor of aconitase, further metabolism, and consequently the energy production, is blocked.

In a somewhat similar manner, amino acid antagonists (e.g., azaserine and fluorophenylalanine) can interfere with the utilization of specific amino acids in the synthesis of proteins.

The energy that is liberated by biochemical oxidation is normally stored in the form of high-energy phosphates. Uncoupling agents such as dinitrophenol interfere with the synthesis of energy-rich phosphates, thus the energy is liberated as heat instead of being stored.

Carriers Carriers such as hemoglobin can be affected by a toxicant through preferential binding. For example, carbon monoxide can bind hemoglobin at the site where oxygen is normally bound. Because of its greater affinity for hemoglobin, it can inactivate hemoglobin, and cause manifestations of oxygen deficiency in tissues.

Oxygen transport can also be impaired by an accumulation of methemoglobin, which is an oxidation product of hemoglobin with no oxygen-binding ability. In normal individuals the trace amount of methemoglobin is readily reduced to hemoglobin. Certain toxicants, such as nitrites and aromatic amines, can enhance the formation of methemoglobin and overwhelm the normal process of its reduction to hemoglobin. People with glucose-6-phosphatase dehydrogenase deficiency have a lower capacity to regenerate hemoglobin from methemoglobin and are thus prone to have methemoglobinemia.

Coenzymes

Coenzymes are essential for the normal function of enzymes. Their levels in the body can be diminished by toxicants that inhibit their synthesis. For example, pyrithiamine can inhibit thiamine kinase, which is responsible for the formation of the coenzyme thiamine pyrophosphate. NADPH can be destroyed in the presence of free radicals, which can be produced by such toxicants as carbon tetrachloride.

Metal-dependent enzymes can be inhibited by chelating agents (e.g., cyanides and dithiocarbamates) through removal of metal coenzymes such as copper and zinc.

Lipids

Peroxidation of polyenoic fatty acids has been suggested as a mechanism of the necrotic action of a number of toxicants, e.g., carbon tetrachloride.

Membrane dissolution can follow contact with organic solvents and amphoteric detergents. Lead ion can increase the fragility of erythrocytes and result in hemolysis. The oxygen-carrying function of hemoglobin is lost after it escapes from the hemolyzed erythrocytes. The ions of mercury and cadmium can complex with phospholipid bases and expand the surface area of the membrane, thereby altering its function.

The general anesthetics ether and halothane as well as many other lipophilic substances can accumulate in the cell membranes and thereby interfere with transport of oxygen and glucose into the cell. The cells of the central nervous system are especially susceptible to a lowering of oxygen tension and glucose level and are therefore among the first to be deleteriously affected by these substances.

Nucleic Acids

Covalent binding between a toxicant (such as alkylating agents) and replicating DNA and RNA can cause serious lesions, e.g., cancer, mutation, teratogenesis. Such toxicants may also exert immuno-suppressive effects (see Chapter 18).

Antimetabolites such as aminopterin and methotrexate may be incorporated into DNA and RNA and then interfere with their replication.

Others

Hypersensitization reactions result from repeated exposure to a particular substance or to its chemically related substances. The latter phenomenon is referred to as cross sensitization. The substance, if it is a large polypeptide, acts as an antigen and stimulates the body to form antibodies. Otherwise, the substance acts as a hapten and combines with proteins in the body to form antigens. The reaction between an antigen and the corresponding antibodies results in the release of histamine, bradykinin, and others. The reaction has a typical pattern irrespective of the nature of the antigen. Photosensitization reaction is somewhat similar except sunlight is also required for its induction.

Corrosive agents such as strong acids and bases can destroy local tissues by precipitating cellular proteins. Irritation of the underlying tissues occurs as a consequence.

Blockade of renal and biliary tubules may follow the precipitation of relatively insoluble toxicants or their metabolites. For example, acetylsulfapyridine, a metabolite of sulfapyridine, may block renal tubules, and harmol glucuronide from harmol may cause cholestasis.

A more detailed discussion on some of the mechanisms of toxic effects is presented by Bridges et al. (1983). Table 4-1 summarizes the various modes of action, representative chemicals, initiating factors, and the early molecular target.

Table 4-1 Types of Chemically Induced Toxicity

	Chemical	Initiating factor	Early molecular target
Enzyme inhibition	parathion	paraxon	cholinesterase
	fluoroacetate	fluorocitrate	aconitase
	dinitrophenol	dinitrophenol	uncouples oxidative phosphorylation
	rotenone	rotenone	inhibits oxidative phosphorylation
Cofactor depletion	galactosamine	UDP galactosamine*	UTP depletion
	ethionine	S-adenosylethionine	adenine/ATP
	menaquinone	semiquinone	NAD(P)H depletion
Receptor interactions	TCDD	TCDD	binding to cytosolic receptor
Physicochemical changes			
Redox	aniline	phenylhydroxylamine	hemoglobin to methemoglobin
Redox	paracetamol	quinoneimine	oxidative damage
Solubility	sulfapyridine	acetylsulfapyridine	precipitation in tubules
Solubility	harmol	harmoglucuronide	biliary cholestasis
Physical damage	silica	silica	lysosomal membranes
Solvation	hexane	hexane	membranes

Source: Bridges et al., 1983.

*UDP and UTP are uridine diphosphate and triphosphate, respectively.

RECEPTORS

Historical Notes

It has long been observed that a number of poisons and toxins exert certain specific biologic effects. To explain such specificity, Paul Ehrlich in 1897 attributed the neutralization of bacterial toxins by antibodies to the presence of specific "side chains" on the antibodies. These side chains would interact with the particular type of toxins.

The concept of a "receptive substance" as the site of action of chemicals was first proposed by John N. Langley. He observed that the effects of nicotine and curare on skeletal muscle were not altered after degeneration of the nerves supplying the muscle, indicating the noninvolvement of the nerve endings as had been believed. Furthermore, the muscular contraction induced by direct stimulation was not influenced by these chemicals. These observations led him to believe that "the poisons do not act on the contractile substances in the muscle, but on other substances in the muscle which may be called "receptive substances" (Langley, 1905). More details on the origins of the receptor theory have been provided by Parascandola (1982).

The existence of a receptive substance proposed in 1905 was only accepted by others after a lapse of more than 30 years. The early users of the concept included Pfeiffer (1948) and Ing (1949). Since then, the concept has greatly facilitated the evolution of pharmacology, especially in relation to the pharmacologic actions and the dose-response relationships of agonists and antagonists of various neurotransmitters. Nevertheless, it has only been in the past 10 years or so that studies of the nature, mechanisms of action, and other aspects of receptors have attracted intensive investigation. That receptors are protein in nature was first suggested by Welsh and Taub (1951) and tentatively demonstrated by Lu (1952).

Chemical Nature

Preliminary Demonstration In the early 1950s, it was generally agreed that in certain organs, such as the ileum, acetylcholine stimulates the smooth muscle via cholinergic receptors, whereas others (e.g., barium chloride) act directly on the muscle. It was also recognized that enzymes have relatively specific substrate requirements; consequently, the chemical nature of a biologically active substance can be deduced by the disappearance of activity after treatment with a particular enzyme. This approach was used, for example, in demonstrating that the posterior pituitary hormones were proteins or polypeptides, because their activities were lost after digestion with trypsin. This conclusion was reached before the hormones could be purified and analyzed.

Using this approach, Lu (1952) showed that the stimulant effect of acetylcholine on isolated rabbit ileum was lost after it was treated with trypsin

(10 mg/100 ml) for 30 min. Conversely, the effect of barium chloride, a direct-acting muscle stimulant, was not altered. On the other hand, chymotrypsin reduced the effects of acetylcholine and barium chloride to the same extent. This finding was interpreted as indicating that chymotrypsin affected the contractile substance of the smooth muscle. As expected, pepsin and inactivated trypsin had no effect on these muscle stimulants.

Isolation and Characterization of Acetylcholine Receptors In the early 1970s, chilinergic receptors (ChR) were solubilized, isolated, and characterized by several groups of investigators. References to their reports are provided by Heilbronn (1976). In general, ChRs were solubilized from appropriate tissues with a surface-active agent such as deoxycholate or non-ionic detergent (e.g., Triton X-100). The most suitable tissue was the electric organ of *Torpedo marmorata*, which contains 100 nmol/kg of ChR. The amino acid composition of ChR was reported by, among others, Heilbronn et al. (1975). They also found that ChR contained 5.4% or 6.0% carbohydrates, consisting of mannose, glucose, and *N*-acetylglucosamine.

Other Receptors *Insulin* receptors have been solubilized from liver and fat-cell membranes with Triton X-100 and extensively studied. The solubilized receptors retained their specific ability to bind insulin. Protein-denaturing agents, such as urea and guanidine, caused a marked loss in insulin-binding activity. Furthermore, trypsin digestion of the fat cells led to a loss of binding ability and biologic responsiveness. These biologic activities could also be reduced by exposing the insulin receptors to β-galactosidase and neuraminidase. These findings thus demonstrate that the insulin receptors are a glycoprotein (Jacobs and Cuatrecasas, 1976).

Cuatrecasas (1971) observed that trypsin at a concentration of 10 μg/ml greatly reduced the biologic activity of the insulin receptor, and at a higher concentration (100 μg/ml), the activity was virtually eliminated. It is interesting to note that the latter concentration is exactly the same as that (10 mg/100 ml) used in abolishing the responsiveness of the cholinergic receptor to acetylcholine (Lu, 1952).

β-Adrenergic receptors have been solubilized from turkey erythrocyte membranes with digitonin. The receptors, isolated from the solution with affinity chromatography, consisted entirely or mainly of proteins.

Categories

Although only a few types of receptors have been isolated, identified, and characterized, many others have been identified and characterized in situ, using pharmacologic, biochemical, and immunologic procedures. The results indicate that receptors have a variety of functions.

Neurotransmitter receptors include the cholinergic (nicotine, located in ganglia and skeletal muscles, and muscarinic in smooth muscles and brain), α- and β-adrenergic, dopamine, opiates (e.g., endorphin), and histamine (H_1 and H_2) receptors.

Hormone receptors are for insulin, cortisone, ACTH, thyrotropin, estrogen, progesterone, angiotensin, glucagon, prostaglandin, and others.

"Drug receptors": certain chemicals such as antidepressants and antitumor agents bind with specific macromolecules that may be considered as receptors. These receptors may well have endogenous messengers (such as endorphins and enkephalins for opiates) but are as yet undiscovered. It has also been suggested that for certain receptors, a physiologic ligand existed at some point in evolution (Poland and Knutsen, 1981).

Mechanism of Action

The receptor functions as the site of biologic system that is able to recognize substances with a specific chemical nature and, after binding with the particular substance, to initiate a certain biologic effect. The major mechanisms of action are as follows.

Adenylate (or Guanylate) Cyclase A common sequence involving this enzyme includes the following: (1) The substance (ligand) binds with the receptor, which then undergoes conformational changes. (2) The ligand-receptor complex causes the regulatory protein to bind with guanosine triphosphate (GTP). (3) This protein-GTP complex activates adenylate cyclase and induces a dissociation of the ligand-receptor complex, thus freeing the receptor for further action. (4) The activated adenylate cyclase (or guanylate cyclase) stimulates the conversion of ATP to cyclic adenosine monophosphate (cAMP) [or to cyclic guanosine monophosphate (cGMP)]. (5) Cyclic AMP (or GMP) acts as a second messenger and amplifier by activating certain protein kinases that phosphorylate proteins, mainly enzymes. (6) The changed enzyme function triggers the biologic effect (Wood, 1982).

Calcium Ion Channel In certain cases, the binding of the ligand to the receptor results in the formation of Ca^{2+} channels, probably through the hydrolysis of phosphatidyl inositol catalyzed by phospholipase. The elevated intracellular Ca^{2+} concentration causes contraction, exocytosis, mitosis, and altered membrane permeability and metabolism.

Berridge (1981) compiled information on the effects of a number of messengers on adenylate cyclase, guanylate cyclase, and calcium gates (see Fig. 4-1).

Receptors in Toxicology

The receptor concept has been valuable in advancing our understanding of certain biochemical, physiologic, and pharmacologic effects, as well as facilitating

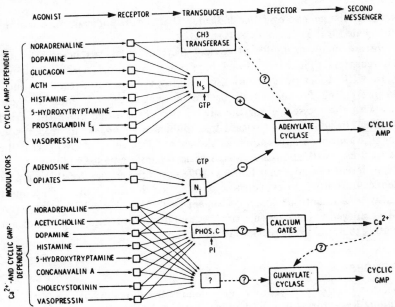

Figure 4-1 Schematic presentation of the signal-processing pathways responsible for generating second messengers. Cyclic AMP-dependent agonists use a GTP-regulatory protein (N_s) to pass information from the receptor to adenylate cyclase. Agonists that act through calcium and cyclic GMP may have access to several transducing systems, including an inhibitory GTP-regulatory protein (N_i); phospholipase C (*Phos. C*), which hydrolyzes phosphatidylinositol (*PI*); and an unknown mechanism that activates guanylate cyclase (from Berridge, 1981).

the developments of drugs. However, it has not played as prominent a role in toxicology. With the advent of molecular toxicology, the use of the receptor concept will undoubtedly aid in the understanding of the mechanism of action of toxicants, as has been pointed out by Campbell (1976). More specifically, Main (1980) noted that the emergence of methods for locating and purifying receptors and the increasing knowledge of the role of receptors in the regulation of body functions are especially useful in this respect.

Poland and Knutson (1982) reviewed the extensive literature on TCDD (2,3,7,8-tetrachlorodibenzo-*p*-dioxin) and related halogenated aromatic hydrocarbons with respect to their toxicity, their ability to induce AHH (aryl hydrocarbon hydroxylase), and their affinity for a cytosol receptor. They suggested that the existence of the receptor could satisfactorily explain the structure-activity data, dose-response curves for AHH induction, and receptor binding in vitro. It was also noted that the concentration of this cytosol receptor is much higher in the liver of C57BL/6 mice than that of DBA/2 mice and that the former strain of mice was much more susceptible than the latter with respect to TCCD-induced thymus involution, teratogenesis, and hepatic porphyria.

Furthermore, the genetic evidence indicated that the *Ah* locus in mice was the structural gene for the cytosol receptor.

There are many examples of toxic effects of chemicals being mediated through receptors that serve normal physiologic functions. Thus, an agonist may cause toxic effect by failing to dissociate from the receptor readily enough, thereby preventing further action of the messenger, and an antagonist can compete with the messenger for the site on the receptor and block the action of the latter. In addition, a toxicant may induce tolerance to its toxicity by reducing the number of receptors, as shown by Costa et al. (1981) with the chronic treatment with an organophosphate acetylcholinesterase inhibitor.

It is of interest to note that Loomis (1978) used the concept of the complex of [chemical-receptor] to explain the existence of thresholds that "there must necessarily be a quantity of chemical agent below which no biological effect would be achieved." The existence of threshold doses for chemicals is important in evaluating their safety, as is elaborated in Chapter 7.

REFERENCES

Berridge, M. J. (1981) Receptors and calcium signalling. In: *Towards Understanding Receptors*. Ed. J. W. Lamble. New York: Elsevier.

Bridges, J. W., Benford, D. J., and Hubbard, S. A. (1983) Mechanisms of toxic injury. *Ann. NY Acad. Sci.* 407:42–63.

Campbell, T. C. (1976) Modern concepts of nutritional status and foreign compound toxicity. In: *New Concepts in Safety Evaluation: Part I*. Eds. M. A. Mehlman, P. E. Shapiro, and H. Blumenthal. Washington, D.C.: Hemisphere.

Costa, L. G., Schwab, B. W., Hand, H., and Murphy, S. D. (1981) Reduced [H^3] quinuclidinyl benzilate binding to muscarinic receptors in disulfoton-tolerant mice. *Toxicol. Appl. Pharmacol.* 60:441–450.

Cuatrecasas, P. (1971) Perturbation of the insulin receptor of isolated fat cells with proteolytic enzymes. *J. Biol. Chem.* 246:6522–6531.

Grice, H. C. (1972) The changing role of pathology in modern safety evaluation. *Crit. Rev. Toxicol.* 1:119–152.

Heilbronn, E. (1976) Neuromuscular transmission after immunization with nicotinic acetylcholine receptor. In: *Motor Innervation*. Ed. S. Thesleff. New York: Academic Press.

Heilbronn, E., Mattsson, C., and Elfman, L. (1975) Biochemical and physical properties of the nicotinic ACh receptor from *Torpedo marmorata*. In: *Properties of Purified Cholinergic and Adrenergic Receptors*, Vol. 37. Ed. M. Wollemann. New York: Elsevier.

Ing, H. R. (1949) The structure-action relationship of the choline group. *Science* 109:264–266.

Jacobs, S., and Cuatrecasas, P. (1976) The insulin receptor. In: *Hormone-Receptor Interaction: Molecular Aspects*. Ed. G. S. Levey. New York: Marcel Dekker.

Kleihues, P., and Cooper, H. K. (1976) Repair excision of alkylated based from DNA *in vivo*. *Oncology* 33:86–88.

Koschier, F. J., Burden, E. J., Brunkhorst, C. S., and Friedman, M. A. (1983) Concentration-dependent elicitation of dermal sensitization in guinea pigs treated with 2,4-toluene diisocyanate. *Toxicol. Appl. Pharmacol.* 67:401–407.

Langley, J. N. (1905) On the reaction of cells and of nerve-endings to certain poisons, chiefly as regards the reaction of striated muscle to nicotine and curari. *J. Physiol.* 33:374–413.

Loomis, T. A. (1978) *Essentials of Toxicology*, 3d ed. Philadelphia: Lea & Febiger.

Lu, F. C. (1952) The effects of proteolytic enzymes on the isolated rabbit intestine. *Br. J. Pharmacol.* 7:624–640.

Main, A. R. (1980) Toxicant-receptor interactions: Fundamental principles. In: *Introduction to Biochemical Toxicology*. Eds. E. Hodgson and F. E. Guthrie. New York: Elsevier.

Mazze, R. I., and Cousins, M. J. (1973) Renal toxicity of anesthetics. *Can. Anaesth. Soc. J.* 20:64–80.

Parascandola, J. (1982) Origins of the receptor theory. In: *Towards Understanding Receptors*. Ed. J. W. Lamble. New York: Elsevier.

Pfieffer, C. C. (1948) Nature and spatial relationship of the prosthetic chemical groups required for maximum muscarinic action. *Science* 107:94–96.

Poland, A., and Knutson, J. C. (1982) 2,3,7,8-Tetrachlorodibenzo-*p*-dioxin and related halogenated aromatic hydrocarbons: Examination of the mechanism of toxicity. *Annu. Rev. Pharmacol. Toxicol.* 22:517–554.

Sharratt, M., and Frazer, A. C. (1963) The sensitivity of function tests in detecting renal damage in the rat. *Toxicol. Appl. Pharmacol.* 5:36–48.

Welsh, J. H., and Taub, R. (1951) The significance of the carbonyl group and ether oxygen in the reaction of acetylcholine with receptor substance. *J. Pharmacol. Exp. Ther.* 103:62–73.

WHO (1978) Chemobiokinetics and metabolism. In: *Environmental Health Criteria 6*. Geneva: World Health Organization.

Wood, A. J. J. (1982) Drug receptor interactions. In: *Drug Anesthesia*. Eds. M. Wood and A. J. J. Wood. Baltimore: Williams & Wilkins.

Zbinden, G. (1976) *Progress in Toxicology*, Vol. 2. Berlin: Springer-Verlag.

ADDITIONAL READINGS

Ariens, E. J., Simonis, A. M., and Offermeier, J. (1976) Classification of toxic effects. In: *Introduction to General Toxicology*. Eds. E. J. Ariens, A. M. Simonis, and J. Offermeier. New York: Academic Press.

Blumberg, P. M., Delcos, B. K., Dunn, J. A., Jaken, S., Leach, K. L., and Yeh, E. (1983) Phorbol ester receptors and the in vitro effects of tumor promoters. *Ann. NY Acad. Sci.* 407:303–315.

Brabec, M. J., and Bernstein, I. A. (1981) Cellular, subcellular, and molecular targets of foreign compounds. In: *Toxicology: Principles and Practice*, Vol. 1. Ed. A. L. Reeves. New York: John Wiley.

Goldstein, A., Aranow, L., and Kalman, S. M. (1974) *Principles of Drug Action*. New York: John Wiley.

Klaassen, C. D., and Doull, J. (1980) Evaluation of safety: Toxic evaluation. In: *Casarett and Doull's Toxicology*. Eds. J. Doull, C. D. Klaassen, and M. O. Amdur. New York: Macmillan.

Miledi, R., and Potter, L. J. (1971) Acetylcholine receptors in muscle fibers. *Nature* 233:599–603.

Chapter 5

Modifying Factors of Toxic Effects

GENERAL REMARKS

While toxicity is an inherent property of a substance, the nature and extent of the toxic manifestations in an organism that is exposed to the substance depend on a variety of factors. The obvious ones are the dose and duration of exposure.

They also include such less obvious host factors as the species and strain of the animal, its sex and age, and its nutritional and hormonal status. Various physical, environmental, and social factors also play a part. In addition, the toxic effect of a chemical may be influenced by simultaneous and consecutive exposure to other chemicals.

The toxic effects may be modified in a number of ways: alterations of the absorption, distribution, and excretion of a chemical; an increase or decrease of its biotransformation; and changes of the sensitivity of the receptor at the target organ.

A clear understanding of the existence of these factors and of their mode of action is important in designing the protocols of toxicologic investigations. It is equally important in evaluating the significance of the toxicologic data and in assessing the safety/risk to humans under specified conditions of exposure.

HOST FACTORS

Species, Strain, and Individual

Differences of toxic effect from one species to another have long been recognized. Knowledge in this field has been used to develop, for example, pesticides, which are more toxic to pests than to humans and other mammals. Among various species of mammals, most effects of toxicants are similar. This fact forms the basis of predicting the toxicity to humans from results obtained in toxicologic studies conducted in other mammals, such as the rat, mouse, dog, rabbit, and monkey. There are, however, notable differences in detoxication mechanisms (Williams, 1974).

Some of the differences can be attributed to variations in detoxication mechanisms. For example, the sleeping time induced in several species of laboratory animals by hexobarbital shows marked differences, which are obviously attributable to the activity of the detoxication enzyme as shown in Table 5-1.

Differences in response to hexobarbital, although less marked, also exist among various strains of mice (Jay, 1955). Other examples include ethylene glycol and aniline. Ethylene glycol is metabolized to oxalic acid, which is responsible for the toxicity, or to carbon dioxide. The magnitude of the toxicity of ethylene glycol in animals is in the following order: cat > rat > rabbit, and this is the same for the extent of oxalic acid production. Aniline is metabolized, in the cat and dog, mainly to o-aminophenol, which is more toxic, but it is metabolized mainly to p-aminophenol in the rat and hamster, which are less susceptible to aniline (Timbrell, 1982).

Differences in bioactivation also account for many dissimilarities of toxicity. A notable example is 2-naphthylamine, which produced bladder tumor in the

Table 5-1 Species Differences in Duration of Action and Metabolism of Hexobarbital. Dose of Barbiturate 50 mg/kg in Dogs, 100 mg/kg in the other Animals

Species	Duration of action (min)	Plasma half-life (min)	Relative enzyme activity [(μg/g)/h)]	Plasma level on awakening (μg/ml)
Mouse	12	19	598	89
Rabbit	49	60	196	57
Rat	90	140	135	64
Dog	315	260	36	19

Source: Quinn et al. 1958. (Copyright © 1958, Pergamon Press, Ltd., Oxford. Reproduced with permission.)

dog and human but not in the rat, rabbit, or guinea pig. Dogs and humans, but not the others, excrete the carcinogenic metabolite 2-naphthyl hydroxylamine (Miller et al., 1964). Acetylaminofluorene (AAF) is carcinogenic to many species of animals but not to the guinea pig. However, the N-hydroxy metabolite of AAF is carcinogenic to all animals including the guinea pig, demonstrating that the difference between the guinea pig and the other animals is not in their response to the toxicant but in the bioactivation (Weisburger and Weisburger, 1973). Many references, e.g., Hucker (1970), provide information on species differences with other chemicals.

Although differences in biotransformation, including bioactivation, account for species variation in susceptibility to a great majority of chemicals, other factors such as absorption, distribution, and excretion also play a part. A number of examples are provided by Timbrell (1982). In addition, variations in physiologic function are important in toxic manifestations in response to such toxicants as squill. This toxic chemical is a good rodenticide because rats cannot vomit, whereas humans and many other mammals can eliminate this poison by vomiting (Doull, 1980). The greater susceptibility of rats to formaldehyde, as compared with mice, was attributed to the findings that rats were less able to reduce minute ventilation on repeated exposure (Chang et al., 1983).

Apart from the variations in susceptibility that exist from one species to another and from one strain to another, there are also variables among individuals of the same species and same strain. While the magnitude of such individual variations is usually relatively small, there are exceptions. This phenomenon has been widely studied among humans. For example, there are "slow inactivators," who are deficient in acetyltransferase. Such individuals acetylate isoniazid only slowly and are thus likely to suffer from peripheral neuropathy resulting from an accumulation of isoniazid. On the other hand, people with more efficient acetyltransferase require larger doses of isoniazid to obtain its therapeutic effect and are thus more likely to suffer from hepatic damage.

Differences in response to succinylcholine provide another example. Individuals with an atypical or a low level of serum cholinesterase may exhibit prolonged muscular relaxation and apnea following an injection of a standard dose of this muscle relaxant.

Glucose-6-phosphate dehydrogenase deficiency and altered stability of reduced glutathione are responsible for hemolytic anemia in subjects exposed to primaquine, antipyrine, and similar agents (Loomis, 1976). A more extensive list of potentially hemolytic chemicals and drugs has been compiled by Calabrese et al. (1979).

Sex, Hormonal Status, and Pregnancy

Male and female animals of the same strain and species usually react to toxicants similarly. There are, however, notable quantitative differences in their susceptibility, especially in the rat. For example, many barbiturates induce more prolonged sleep in female rats than in males. The shorter duration of action of hexobarbital in male rats is related to the higher activity of the liver microsomal enzymes to hydroxylate this chemical. This higher activity can be reduced by castration or pretreatment with estrogen. Similarly, male rats demethylate aminopyrine and acetylate sulfanilamide faster than females, and the males are thus less susceptible.

Female rats are also more susceptible than the males to such organophosphorous insecticides as azinphosmethyl and parathion. Castration and hormone treatments reverse this difference. Furthermore, weanling rats of both sexes are equally susceptible to these toxicants. However, unlike hexobarbital, parathion is metabolized more rapidly in the female rat than in the male. This faster metabolism of parathion results in a higher concentration of its metabolite, paraoxon, which is more toxic than the parent compound. This higher toxicity resulting from greater bioactivation in female rats, compared to males, is also true with aldrin and heptachlor, which undergo epoxidation. The female rat is also more susceptible to warfarin and strychnine. On the other hand, male rats are more susceptible than females to ergot and lead.

Differences in susceptibility between the sexes are also seen with other chemicals. For example, chloroform is acutely nephrotoxic in the male mouse but not in the females. Castration or the administration of estrogens reduces this effect in the males, and treatment with androgens enhances susceptibility to chloroform in the females. The greater susceptibility of male mice was explained on the basis of a much higher concentration of cytochrome P-450 (Smith et al., 1983). Nicotine is also more toxic to the male mouse, and digoxin is more toxic to the male dog. However, the female cat is more susceptible to dinitrophenol and the female rabbit is more so to benzene.

Imbalances of non-sex hormones can also alter the susceptibility of animals to toxicants. Hyperthyroidism, hyperinsulinism, adrenalectomy, and stimulation of the pituitary-adrenal axis have all been shown to be capable of modifying the effects of certain toxicants (Dauterman, 1980; Doull, 1980).

There is some evidence that the pregnant rat (Ivankovic, 1969) is more susceptible to the carcinogenic activity of ethylnitrosourea. Highly malignant tumors, apparently of trophoblastic origin, developed in these animals and were rapidly fatal.

Age

It has long been recognized that neonates and very young animals in general are more susceptible to toxicants such as morphine. For a great majority of toxicants, the young are 1.5–10 times more susceptible than adults (Goldenthal, 1971).

The available information indicates that the greater susceptibility of the young animals to many toxicants can be attributed to deficiencies of various detoxication enzyme systems (Dauterman, 1980). Both phase I and phase II reactions may be responsible. For example, hexobarbital at a dose of 10 mg/kg induced a sleeping time of longer than 360 min in 1-day-old mice compared to 27 min in the 21-day-old. The proportion of hexobarbital metabolized by oxidation in 3 hours in these animals was 0% and 21–33%, respectively (Jondorf et al., 1959). On the other hand, chloramphenicol is excreted mainly as a glucuronide conjugate. When a dose of 50 mg/kg was given to 1- or 2-day-old infants, the blood levels were 15 μg/ml or higher over a period of 48 hours. In contrast, children aged 1–11 years maintained such blood levels for only 12 hours (Weiss et al., 1966).

However, not all chemicals are more toxic to the young. Certain substances, notably CNS stimulants, are much less toxic to neonates. Lu et al. (1965) reported that the LD_{50} of DDT was more than 20 times greater in newborn rats than in adults, in sharp contrast to the effect of age on malathion (Table 5-2). This insensitivity to the toxicity of DDT may be significant in assessing the potential risk of this pesticide, because of the very much larger intake in young babies via breast feeding and cow's milk, especially on the unit body weight basis.

The effect of age on the susceptibility to other CNS stimulants, including other organochlorine insecticides, appears less marked (generally in the range of 2–10 times). Most organophosphorous pesticides are more toxic to the young; Schradan (octamethyl pyrophosphoramide) and phenylthiourea are notable exceptions (Brodeur and DuBois, 1963).

Table 5-2 Effect of Age on Acute Toxicity of Malathion, DDT, and Dieldrin in Rats

Pesticide	Age	LD_{50} (mg/kg) with 95% confidence limits
Malathion	Newborn	134.4 (94.0–190.8)
	Pre-weaning	925.5 (679.0–1261.0)
	Adult	3697.0 (3179.0–4251.0)
DDT	Newborn	>4000.0
	Pre-weaning	437.8 (346.3–553.9)
	Weaning	355.2 (317.2–397.8)
	Adult	194.5 (158.7–238.3)
	Middle-aged	235.8 (208.0–267.4)
Dieldrin	Newborn	167.8 (140.8–200.0)
	Pre-weaning	24.9 (19.7–31.5)
	Adult	37.0 (27.4–50.1)

Source: Lu et al. (1965). (Copyright © 1965, Pergamon Press Ltd., Oxford, Reproduce with permission.)

Apart from differences in biotransformation, other factors also play a role. For example, a lower susceptibility at the receptor has been found to be the reason for the relative insensitivity of young rats to DDT (Henderson and Woolley, 1969).

Certain toxicants are absorbed to a greater extent by the young than by the adult. For example, young children absorb four to five times more lead than adults (McCabe, 1979) and 20 times more cadmium (Sasser and Jarbor, 1977). The greater susceptibility of the young to morphine is attributable to a less efficient blood-brain barrier, as is vividly illustrated in Fig. 5-1 (Kupferberg and Way, 1963). Penicillin and tetracycline are excreted more slowly and hence are more toxic in the young (Lu, 1970). Ouabain is about 40 times more toxic in the newborn than in the adult rat because the adult rat's liver is much more efficient in removing this cardiac glycoside from the plasma. The higher incidence of methemoglobinemia in young infants has been explained on the basis that their lower gastric acidity allows upward migration of intestinal microbial flora and the reduction of nitrates to a greater extent. Furthermore, they have a higher proportion of fetal hemoglobin, which is more readily oxidized to methemoglobin (WHO, 1977).

There is evidence that the newborn is more susceptible to such carcinogens as aflatoxin B_1. Furthermore, the fetuses, but not the embryos, of rodents are much more acceptible. For example, there was a 50-fold increase in the potency of ethylnitrosourea. This is also true with nonhuman primates, except the

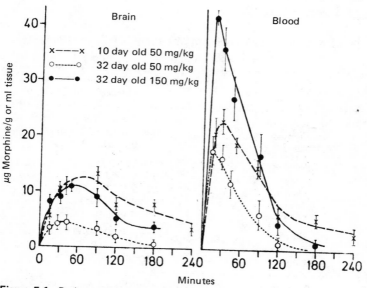

Figure 5-1 Brain and blood levels of free morphine at specific time intervals after intraperitoneal injections of morphine. Bracketed vertical lines show the standard error, using four animals per point (from Kupferberg, H. J., and Way, E. I., 1963).

maximal effects occur during the first third of gestation. If this is true with human fetuses, then they may be exposed to carcinogens before the mothers are aware of their pregnancies (Rice, 1979).

Old animals and humans are also more susceptible to certain chemicals. This problem has not been studied as extensively as in the young. However, the available evidence indicates that the aged patients are generally more sensitive to many drugs. The possible mechanisms include reduced biotransformations and an impaired renal excretion. In addition, the distribution of chemicals in the body may also be altered because of increased body fat and decreased body water (Jarvik et al., 1981).

Nutritional Status

The principal biotransformation of toxicants is catalyzed by the microsomal mixed-function oxidase system (MFO). A deficiency of essential fatty acids generally depresses MFO activities. This is also true with protein deficiency. The decreased MFO has different effects on the toxicity of chemicals. For example, hexobarbital and aminopyrine are detoxicated by these enzymes and are thus more toxic to male rats and mice with these nutrient deficiencies. On the other hand, the toxicities of alfatoxin, carbon tetrachloride, and heptachlor are lower in such animals because of their depressed bioactivation of these toxicants. Rats fed low-protein diets were 2–26 times more sensitive to a variety of pesticides (Boyd, 1972). MFO activities are decreased in animals fed high levels of sugar.

A number of carcinogenesis studies have demonstrated that restriction of food intake decreases tumor yield. Deficiency of protein generally lowers tumorigenicity of carcinogens, such as aflatoxin B_1 and dimethylnitrosamine. The importance of diet on carcinogenesis is further demonstrated by the fact that rats and mice fed diets rich in fats have higher tumor incidences compared to those that are given a restricted diet.

Vitamin A deficiency depressed the MFO. In general, this is also true with deficiencies of vitamins C and E. But thiamine deficiency has the opposite effect. Vitamin A deficiency, in addition, increases the susceptibility of the respiratory tract to carcinogens (Nettesheim et al., 1979).

Some foods contain appreciable amounts of chemicals that are strong inducers of the MFO, e.g., safrole, flavones, xanthines, and indoles. In addition, potent inducers such as DDT and polychlorinated biphenyls (PCB) are present as contaminants in many foods.

For additional details and literature citations, see articles by Campbell (1976), Dauterman (1980), and Parke and Ioannides (1982).

Diseases

The liver is the main organ wherein biotransformation of chemicals takes place. Such diseases as acute and chronic hepatitis, cirrhosis of the liver, and hepatic necrosis often decrease the biotransformation. The microsomal and nonmicrosomal enzyme systems as well as the phase II reactions may be involved.

Renal diseases may also affect the toxic manifestations of chemicals. This effect stems from disturbances of the excretory and metabolic functions of the kidney. Heart diseases, when severe, can increase the toxicity of chemicals by impairing the hepatic and renal circulation, thus affecting the metabolic and excretory functions of these organs.

Examples of chemicals the toxicities of which are affected by diseases of these organs are given by Dauterman (1980) and Timbrell (1982).

ENVIRONMENTAL FACTORS

Physical Factors

Changes in temperature may alter the toxicity. For example, colchicine and digitalis are more toxic to the rat than to the frog. But their toxicity to the frog can be increased by raising the environmental temperature. The duration of the response, however, is shorter when the temperature is higher. The effect of environmental temperature on the magnitude and duration of the response is apparently related to the temperature-dependent biochemical reactions responsible for the effect and for the biotransformation of the chemical.

Interest in the effect of barometric pressure on the toxicity of chemicals stems from human exposure to them in space and in saturation diving vehicles. At high altitudes, the toxicity of digitalis and strychnine is decreases whereas that of amphetamine is increased. The influence of changes in barometric pressure on the toxicity of chemicals seems attributable mainly, if not entirely, to the altered oxygen tension rather than to a direct pressure effect.

Whole-body irradiation increases the toxicity of CNS stimulants but decreases that of CNS depressants. However, it has no effect on analgesics such as morphine. More details and literature citations have been provided by Doull (1980).

The effects of toxicants often show a diurnal pattern that is mainly related to the light cycle. In the rat and the mouse, the activities of cytochrome P-450 are the greatest at the beginning of the dark phase.

Social Factors

It is well known that animal husbandry and a variety of social factors can modify the toxicities of chemicals: the handling of the animals, the housing (singly or in groups), the types of cage, and bedding materials are all important factors. Some examples of the influence of environmental factors on toxicity are given in Chapter 8.

CHEMICAL INTERACTION

Types of Interaction

The toxicity of a chemical in an organism may be increased or decreased by a simultaneous or consecutive exposure to another chemical. If the combined effect is equal to the sum of the effect of each substance given alone, the interaction is considered to be *additive*, e.g., combinations of most organophosphorous pesticides on cholinesterase activity. If the combined effect is greater than the sum, the interaction is considered to be *synergistic*, e.g., carbon tetrachloride and ethanol on the liver. The term *potentiation* is used to describe the situation in which the toxicity of a substance on an organ is markedly increased by another substance that alone has no toxic effect on that organ. For example, ispropanol has no effect on the liver, but it can increase considerably the hepatotoxicity of carbon tetrachloride.

The exposure of an organism to a chemical may reduce the toxicity of another. *Chemical antagonism* denotes the situation wherein a chemical reaction takes place and produces a less toxic product, e.g., chelation of heavy metals by dimercaprol. *Functional antagonism* exists when two chemicals produce opposite effects on the same physiologic parameters, e.g., the counteraction between CNS stimulants and depressants. *Competitive antagonism* exists when the agonist and antagonist act on the same receptor, e.g., the blockade of the effects of nicotine on ganglia by ganglionic blocking agents. *Noncompetitive antagonism* exists when the toxic effect of a chemical is blocked by another with a nonspecific action, namely, not occupying the same receptor, e.g., the reduction of the toxicity of cholinesterase inhibitors by atropine.

Mechanism of Action

Chemical interactions are achieved through a variety of mechanisms. For instance, nitrites and certain amines can react in the stomach to form nitrosamines, the majority of which are potent carcinogens, and thus greatly increase the toxicity. On the other hand, the action of many antidotes is based on their interaction with the toxicants; for example, thiosulfate is used in cases of cyanide poisoning. Furthermore, a chemical may displace another from its binding site on plasma protein and thereby increase its effective concentration. A chemical may modify the renal excretion of weak acids and weak bases by altering the pH of urine. Competition for the same renal transport system by one chemical can hinder the excretion of another.

An important type of interaction involves the binding of chemicals with their specific receptors. An antagonist blocks the action of an agonist, such as a neurotransmitter or a hormone, by preventing the binding of the agonist to the receptor. The concepts that have been proposed to explain their effects include the following:

1 There are accessory receptor sites for the competitive antagonists, and an allosteric interaction exists between agonist and antagonist, each binding to its own receptor site on the receptor molecule. The binding of an agonist excludes the binding of an antagonist to the same receptor and vice versa.

2 The receptor occurs in two forms, the activated and nonactivated, which are in dynamic equilibrium. The agonists stabilize the receptor in the activated form, whereas the antagonists stabilize the nonactivated form (Ariens and De Miranda, 1979).

Another important type of interaction results from alterations of the biotransformation of a chemical by another. Some chemicals are *inducers* of microsomal and nonmicrosomal enzymes. They augment the activities of these enzymes, perhaps mainly by de novo synthesis, a fact that is consistent with the finding that repeated administrations are necessary. The common inducers include phenobarbital, 3-methylcholanthrene (3-MC), PCB, DDT, and BaP. The inducers may lower the toxicity of other chemicals by accelerating their detoxication. For example, pretreatment with phenobarbital shortens the sleeping time induced by hexobarbital and the paralysis induced by zoxazolamine. Such pretreatment also reduces the plasma level of aflatoxins (Wong et al., 1981). In addition, 3-MC pretreatment greatly reduces the liver necrosis produced by bromobenzene, probably by increasing the activity of the epoxide hydrase. On the other hand, pretreatment with phenobarbital augments the toxicity of acetaminophen and bromobenzene, apparently by increasing the toxic metabolites formed (Mazel and Pessayre, 1976; Timbrell, 1982). Repeated administration of a chemical may induce its metabolizing enzymes, as has been shown with vinyl chloride (Du et al., 1982).

4 Piperonyl butoxide, isoniazid, and SKF 525A and related chemicals are *inhibotors* of various microsomal and nonmicrosomal drug-metabolizing enzymes. For instance, piperonyl butoxide increases the toxicity of pyrethrum in insects by inhibiting their MFO that detoxifies this insecticide. Isoniazid, when taken along with diphenylhydantoin, lengthens the plasma half-life of the antiepileptic drug and increases its toxicity. Iproniazid inhibits monoamine oxidase and increases the cardiovascular effects of tyramine, which is found in cheese and which is normally readily metabolized by the oxidase (Timbrell, 1982).

The action of *promoters* such as phorbol esters in promoting the activity of benzo[a]pyrene and other carcinogens represents a classic type of chemical interaction. The interaction between cigarette smoking and exposure to asbestos in causing various types of respiratory lesions has great public health and social significance.

Interaction as Toxicologic Tools

Not only are studies on chemical interaction conducted to determine the effects of combinations of chemicals, but the data thereof are useful in assessing health hazards associated with exposures to such combinations. These studies are also done to elucidate the nature and the mode of action of the toxicity of a chemical by the administration of another as well as to bring out weak or latent effects of chemicals. Examples of such studies are given in the chapters in Part II and Part III of this book.

REFERENCES

Ariens, E. J., and De Miranda, J. F. R. (1979) The receptor concept: Recent experimental and theoretical developments. In: *Recent Advances in Receptor Chemistry*. Eds. F. Gualtieri, M. Giannella, and C. Lelchiore. New York: Elsevier.

Boyd, E. M. (1972) *Protein Deficiency and Pesticide Toxicity*. Springfield, Ill.: Charles C. Thomas.

Brodeur, J., and DuBois, K. P. (1963) Comparison of acute toxicity of anticholinesterase insecticides to weanling and adult male rats. *Proc. Soc. Exp. Biol. Med.* 114:509–511.

Calabrese, E. J., Moore, G., and Brown, R. (1979) Effects of environmental oxidant stressors on individuals with a G-6-PD deficiency with particular reference to an animal model. *Environ. Health Persp.* 29:49–55.

Campbell, T. C. (1976) Modern concepts in nutritional status and foreign compound toxicity. In: *New Concepts in Safety Evaluation: Part I*. Eds. M. A. Mehlman, R. E. Shaprio, and H. Blumenthal. Washington, D.C.: Hemisphere.

Chang, J. C. F., Cross, F. A., Svenberg, J. A., and Barrow, C. S. (1983) Nasal cavity deposition, histopathology and cell proliferation after single or repeated formaldehyde exposures in B6C3F1 mice and F-344 rats. *Toxicol. Appl. Pharmacol.* 68:161–176.

Dauterman, W. C. (1980) Physiological factors affecting metabolism of xenobiotics. In: *Introduction to Biochemical Toxicology*. Eds. E. Hodgson and F. E. Guthrie. New York: Elsevier.

Doull, J. (1980) Factors influencing toxicology. In: *Casarett and Doull's Toxicology*. Eds. J. Doull, C. D. Klaassen, and M. O. Amdur. New York: Macmillan.

Du, J. T., Tseng, M. T., and Tamburro, C. H. (1982) The effect of repeated vinyl chloride exposure on rat hepatic metabolizing enzymes. *Toxicol. Appl. Pharmacol.* 62:1–10.

Goldenthal, E. I. (1971) A compilation of LD_{50} values in newborn and adult animals. *Toxicol. Appl. Pharmacol.* 18:185–207.

Henderson, G. L., and Woolley, D. A. (1969) Studies on the relative insensitivity of the immature rat to the neurotoxic effects of DDT. *J. Pharmacol. Exp. Ther.* 170:173–180.

Hucker, H. B. (1970) Species differences in drug metabolism. *Ann. Rev. Pharmacol.* 10:99–118.

Ivankovic, S. (1969) Erzeugung von Genital-krebs bei trachtigen Ratten. *Arzneimittel Forsch.* 19:1040.

Jarvik, L. F., Greenblatt, D. J., and Harman, D. (1981) *Clinical Pharmacology and the Aged Patient*. New York: Raven Press.

Jay, G. E., Jr. (1955) Variation in response of various mouse strains to hexo-barbital (Evipal). *Proc. Soc. Exp. Biol. Med.* 90:378–380.

Jondorf, W. R., Maickel, R. P., and Brodie, B. B. (1959) Inability of newborn mice and guinea pigs to metabolize drugs. *Biochem. Pharmacol.* 1:352–354.

Kupferberg, H. J., and Way, E. L. (1963) Pharmacologic basis for the increased sensitivity of the newborn rat to morphine. *J. Pharmacol. Exp. Ther.* 141: 105–112.

Loomis, T. A. (1976) *Essentials of Toxicology*, 3d ed. Philadelphia: Lea & Febiger.

Lu, F. C., Jessup, D. C., and Lavellee, A. (1965) Toxicity of pesticides in young versus adult rats. *Food Cosmet. Toxicol.* 3:591–596.

Lu, F. C. (1970) Significance of age of test animals in food additive evaluation. In: *Metabolic Aspects of Food Safety*. Ed. F. J. C. Roe. Oxford: Blackwell Scientific.

McCabe, E. B. (1979) Age and sensitivity to lead toxicity: A review. *Environ. Health Persp.* 29:29–33.

Mazel, P., and Pessayre, D. (1976) Significance of metabolite-mediated toxicities in the safety evaluation of drugs and chemicals. In: *New Concepts in Safety Evaluation: Part I*. Eds. M. A. Mehlman, R. E. Shapiro, and H. Blumenthal. Washington, D.C.: Hemisphere.

Miller, E. C., Miller, J. H., and Enomotor, M. (1964) The comparative carcino-genetics of 2-acetylaminofluorene and its *N*-hydroxy metabolite in mice, hamsters and guinea pigs. *Cancer Res.* 24:2018–2032.

Nettesheim, P., Snyder, C., and Kim, J. C. S. (1979) Vitamin A and the sus-ceptibility of respiratory tract tissues to carcinogenic insult. *Environ. Health Perspect.* 29:89–93.

Park, D. V., and Ioannides, C. (1981) The role of nutrition in toxicology. *Annu. Rev. Nutr.* 1:207–234.

Quinn, G. P., Axelrod, J., and Brodie, B. B. (1958) Species, strain and sex dif-ferences in metabolism of hexobarbitone, amidopyrine, antipyrine and aniline. *Biochem. Pharmacol.* 1:152–159.

Rice, J. M. (1979) Perinatal period and pregnancy: Intervals of high risk for chemical carcinogens. *Environ. Health Perspect.* 29:23–27.

Sasser, L. B., and Jarbor, G. E. (1977) Intestinal absorption and retention of cadmium in neonatal rat. *Toxicol. Appl. Pharmacol.* 41:423–431.

Smith, J. H., Maita, K., Adler, V., Schacht, T., Sleight, S. D., and Hook, J. B. (1983) Effect of sex hormone status on chloroform nephrotoxicity and renal drug metabolizing enzymes. *Toxicol. Lett.* 28(Suppl. 1):23.

Timbrell, J. A. (1982) *Principles of Biochemical Toxicology*. London: Taylor & Francis.

Weisburger, J. H., and Weisburger, E. K. (1973) Biochemical formation and pharmacological, toxicological and pathological properties of hydroxyl-amines and hydroxamic acids. *Pharmacol. Rev.* 25:1–66.

Weiss, C. G., Glazko, A. J., and Weston, A. (1960) Chloramphenicol in the newborn infant. A physicologic explanation of its toxicity when given in excessive doses. *N. Engl. J. Med.* 262:787–794.

WHO (1977) Nitrates, Nitrites and *N*-Nitroso Compounds. *Environmental Health Criteria 5*. Geneva: World Health Organization.

Williams, R. T. (1974) Inter-species variations in the metabolism of xenobiotics. *Biochem. Soc. Trans.* 2:359–377.

Wong, Z. A., Wei, Ching-I, Rice, D. W., and Hsieh, D.P.H. (1981) Effects of phenobarbital pretreatment on the metabolism and toxicokinetics of aflatoxin B_1 in the rhesus monkey. *Toxicol. Appl. Pharmacol.* 60:387–397.

ADDITIONAL READING

Kluwe, W. M., and Hook, J. B. (1981) Potentiation of acute chloroform nephrotoxicity by the glutathione depletor diethyl maleate and protection by the microsomal enzyme inhibitor piperonyl butoxide. *Toxicol. Appl. Pharmacol.* 59:457–466.

Chapter 6

Acquisition of Data

INTRODUCTION

The toxicity of a chemical can manifest, as outlined in Chapter 4, in a variety of ways. Furthermore, the toxic effects can be modified by many host and environmental factors (Chapter 5). Therefore, for a satisfactory toxicologic evaluation, sufficient, relevant toxicity data must be acquired. Such data are, as a rule, generated from various test systems using many types of examinations and measurements. These topics will be elaborated in the chapters in Part II, "Testing Procedures," and in those in Part III, "Target Organs." There are, however, a number of items that merit a general consideration.

TOXICITY DATA FROM HUMANS

Since the purpose of the toxicologic evaluation is to assess the safety/risk of chemicals in humans, the data ideally should be obtained from humans. However, it is inadvisable to wait for the development of human data for the following reasons:

1 The large number of toxicants whose risks to humans need evaluation
2 The difficulty in distinguishing the effects of the many potentially
hazardous substances to which humans are simultaneously exposed.
3 The prolonged latency after an exposure or the long duration of continual exposure that is required for certain toxic effects to manifest clinically.
4 The impracticality of finding sufficient numbers of exposed and control
people to make valid comparisons in terms of health status, especially with
respect to insidious and subtle effects

Nevertheless, certain information on the effects of chemicals in humans can be
acquired by various means. These include medical surveillance of workers exposed to specific chemicals, epidemiologic studies of special segments of the
population, and clinical studies of patients overdosed with medications as well
as those accidentally or intentionally exposed to large amounts of toxic chemicals. Furthermore, under specific conditions, limited metabolic studies may be
conducted (National Academy of Sciences, 1965). Such information is useful in
establishing the profile of toxicity of chemicals, e.g., in revealing effects specific
to humans, in facilitating appropriate antidotal and other therapy, and in providing a sound basis for extrapolating animal data to humans.

TOXICOLOGIC STUDIES IN ANIMALS

In general, the effects of a toxicant elicited in laboratory animals can be expected to occur in humans under appropriate conditions. Consequently, studies
in laboratory animals have become a main source of toxicologic data.

Limitations and Advantages

As noted in previous chapters, the toxic effects of a chemical may vary from one
species to another and are subject to the influence of many modifying factors.
In extrapolating the results obtained in animals to humans, any knowledge of
species difference and influence of modifying factors is taken into account. But
there remains considerable uncertainty about the degree of confidence of the
predicted toxicity in humans. The confidence can usually be increased by the
following action:

1 The use of several species of animals
2 A thorough investigation of the pattern and rate of biotransformation of
the chemical in these species and in humans
3 Incorporating into the protocols of toxicologic studies a set of conditions
that resembles, as closely as feasible, the human exposure situation

On the positive side of animal studies, one should note that it is usually
feasible in animal studies to employ one or more relatively high doses that will

induce overt signs of toxicity. These signs will help to pinpoint the target organ and the specific effect, which can then be critically examined in animals treated with lower doses. The use of such high doses can also partly obviate the need for placing very large numbers of animals in the studies.

Furthermore, it is also feasible in animal studies to rigidly control the experimental conditions and to determine the effects of a toxicant by taking a great variety of measurements, including pathologic studies. Examination for morphologic changes is significant in view of the fact that these changes may occur in the absence of alterations in biochemical and functional parameters. All these points, although important, are difficult to implement in studies in humans.

Types of Studies

In view of the diversity of toxic effects, a variety of studies are in use. These involve either intact animals or isolated organs or cells. With intact animals, rats and mice are the most commonly used. Others include dogs, monkeys, hamsters, and guinea pigs. The exposure of the animals to the chemicals may be on one occasion only or repeated either during a limited period of time or over the entire life span.

The nature of toxic effects often varies with the dose. For instance, as the dose of a barbiturate increases, the effects progress through no observable effect, to mild sedation, to loss of righting reflex (sleep), to death. Furthermore, because of differences of individual susceptibility, not all animals exposed to the same dose will respond the same way. Based on the doses, the effects and the responses (incidences), simple statistical analyses will yield information on the dose-effect and dose-response relationships.

Occasionally, such quantitative information can be derived from human data. For example, with increasing intakes of methyl mercury, there were paresthesia, ataxia, dysarthria, deafness, and death, as well as greater proportions of individuals manifesting these effects (Bakir et al., 1973). Figure 6-1 shows graphically both the dose-response and dose-effect relationships among individuals exposed to various amounts of methyl mercury.

In toxicity studies, many types of examinations and measurements can be made. These include gross observations, instrumental examinations of physiologic functions, light and electron microscopy, and various biochemical studies. As a rule, general studies are carried out on intact animals. These are followed by detailed studies on the target organ(s) and/or special studies such as teratogenesis and mutagenesis. Apart from intact mammals and isolated organs and cells, other biologic systems (e.g., microorganisms, insects, and such birds as the duck and Japanese quail) are also used for special purposes.

SELECTION OF CHEMICALS FOR TESTING

Ideally, all new chemicals should be toxicologically tested before manufacture and sale. But, because of the very large number of chemicals that may pose a

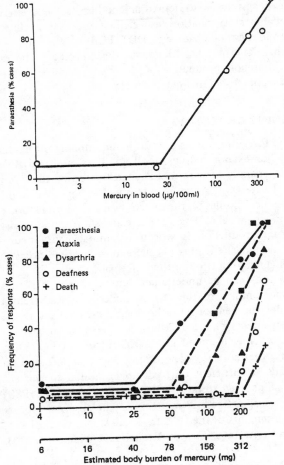

Figure 6-1 Dose-response and dose-effect relationship of humans exposed to methyl mercury. Upper portion shows an increase in response (paraesthesia) as dose (mercury in blood) increases. Lower portion shows that increase of dose (body burden of mercury estimated according to two different procesures) is associated with not only greater responses but also additional effects (from WHO, 1976).

health hazard to humans and the limited facilities and personnel, priority must be assigned in the selection of chemicals for testing. High priority is usually assigned to chemicals according to the following criteria:

1   Chemicals that are directly consumed by humans, such as drugs and food additives
2   Chemicals that are suspected of capable of causing serious and irreversible toxicity, e.g., carcinoma, CNS damages

3 Chemicals that are persistent in the environment because of their resistance to degradation and biotransformation, especially those that are likely to undergo biomagnification in the food chain, e.g., DDT, PCB

4 Chemicals to which a large number of people are expected to be exposed, such as chemicals in household products

5 Chemicals that are manufactured in large quantities

THE EXTENT AND PLANNING OF TESTING

The criteria described in the foregoing are also useful in determining the extent of testing that is required. For example, drugs, food additives, and pesticides that leave residues in food generally require more extensive testing than, say, an ingredient of a household detergent. A "more extensive" testing usually consists of a series of (1) biochemical studies on the metabolism and biotransformation of the toxicant and its biochemical effects, (2) acute and short-term toxicity studies, (3) special studies on reproduction, teratogenicity, mutagenicity, neurotoxicity, potentiation, etc., as indicated, plus (4) the exposure of at least two species of animals for at least a major portion of their life span.

In practice, not all the tests can be undertaken simultaneously. It is thus important to ensure a proper phasing of the various toxicologic studies of a chemical in relation to the development of its technological use data and to the generation of data on health effects on occupational workers and on environmental impact. A proposed scheme, included in a WHO document (1978), is reproduced as Table 6-1. Furthermore, in view of the fact that information gathered in certain tests may be sufficient on toxicologic ground to warrant discontinuation of a series of planned tests, the Food Safety Council (1980) recently proposed a "safety decision tree." A summary of the proposal appears in Fig. 6-2. To meet the requirements of the U.S. Toxic Substance Control Act, a chemical firm has described its testing scheme (Attallah and Whitacre, 1980).

THE STORY OF SACCHARIN

The requirements for the testing of a specific chemical may change over the years. As a result, the toxicologic assessment of a chemical may change from "acceptable" to "unacceptable" and to "uncertain." A case in point is the evolution of saccharin testing. Saccharin was discovered in 1879 and used as a sweetener shortly thereafter.

Early information on its safety consisted of the following data:

1 Low acute toxicity (LD_{50} in animals falling in the range of 5–17.5 g/kg)

2 Biochemically inert, being excreted unchanged via the urine

3 Lack of ill effects in volunteers taking up to 4.8 g a day for up to 5 months.

Table 6-1 Extent of Toxicologic Evaluation Required in Relation to Technological Process Development

Stages of technological development	Stages of toxicologic evaluation	Toxicologic studies
1. Theoretical concept and process flow diagram	Preliminary toxicologic assessment	Analysis of literature data on toxicity hazards of raw materials, reagents, catalyzers, semiproducts and additives Assessment of toxicologic parameters on the basis of metabolic analogies, persistence, the relationship between chemical structure, chemical and physical properties, and biological activity. Interpolation and extrapolation in homologous series
2. Laboratory development of the technological process	Acute toxicity	Acute and subacute experiments on animals. Toxicologic evaluation of technological unit processes
3. Pilot plant stage	Subacute toxicity	Subacute toxicity experiments on animals. Studies of delayed effects. Medical examination of workers
	Detailed toxicologic evaluation	Chronic toxicity studies and, when indicated, effects on reproduction, carcinogenicity, mutagenicity. Formulation of medical and industrial hygiene requirements for full-scale production
4. Design of industrial scale process	Additional studies	Studies of the mechanism of action, early and differential diagnosis, experimental therapy
5. Production and use of chemicals	Field studies	Assessment of working and environmental conditions and of health status of workers and general population Epidemiologic studies Clinical evaluation of experimental prophylactic, diagnostic and therapeutic methods Adjustment and correction of requirements for health and environmental protection

Source: WHO, 1978.

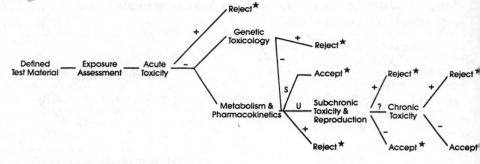

+ = presents socially unacceptable risk
− = does not present a socially unacceptable risk
S = metabolites known and safe
U = metabolites unknown or of doubtful safety
? = decision requires more evidence
★ = see Summary, page 4.

Figure 6-2 Safety decision tree. For further information regarding the last footnote, see text or the original report. (Reprinted with permission from *Food Cosmet. Toxicol.*, Vol. 16, Suppl. 2. Food Safety Council, Proposed system for food safety assessment. Copyright © 1980, Pergamon Press, Ltd.)

Its safety was further demonstrated by two long-term feeding studies, reported in 1923 and 1951, respectively.

Data on Its Carcinogenicity

The confidence in its safety was not shaken in spite of two special carcinogenicity tests done in the 1950s, which yielded weakly positive results. The tests consisted of (1) applying saccharin to the skin followed by croton oil and (2) implanting saccharin in paraffin wax pellets in the urinary bladder in mice. The tests were considered inappropriate for the evaluation of a chemical that is to be taken orally.

In the 1960s, more carcinogenicity tests were conducted. These were done because of the marked increase in the consumption of this artificial sweetener (estimated consumption in United States in 1953: 21,000 pounds; 1963; 2.5 million pounds) and, perhaps more importantly, because of the report that another artificial sweetener, Dulcin (4-ethoxyphenylurea), was shown to be a potent carcinogen, although three previous tests had all yielded negative results. In one of the saccharin tests, up to 5% in the diet had no effect on the tumor incidence. In the other, mixtures of saccharin and cyclamates, in proportions of 1:9, were incorporated in the feed at such levels that the intake was up to 2500 mg/kg body weight. Some of these rats developed bladder tumors. As a result of this study (Price et al., 1970) and other findings, such as that cyclamate was metabolizable to cyclohexylamine, FDA banned cyclamates but left saccharin on the market. A number of other countries followed suit.

Continuing Doubt About Saccharin Safety

The Price paper prompted many further toxicologic studies, using different strains of rats and mice. Still others attempted to assess the effect of saccharin on the tumor yield of known carcinogens. The results from these studies were inconclusive: The role of other factors in the development of bladder tumors was not ruled out. These factors included bladder parasites, calculi, urinary pH, and impurities. One major impurity was OTS (ortho-toluenesulfonamide), which was present in relatively high concentration in some studies that yielded positive results. A comprehensive study was then undertaken by the Canadian government laboratory to investigate the carcinogenicity of OTS in rats, using several dose levels, in both sexes, in the parent and first-generation offspring, and with the urinary pH, bladder parasites, and calculi controlled. OTS proved to be noncarcinogenic in these animals, but saccharin, which was included as a control, produced a few bladder tumors, mainly in the males. The offspring were more susceptible than the parent generation. As a result of these findings, the Canadian and US authorities suspended the sale of saccharin as a food additive.

Along with these carcinogenicity tests, a number of epidemiologic studies were undertaken. Most of these showed no correlation between the consumption of saccharin and the incidence of bladder tumor, but a few others showed a slight increase of the bladder tumor risk among male saccharin consumers. Many short-term mutagenicity tests were carried out. The results were inconclusive. Additional details and references are included in the International Agency on Research and Cancer report (1980) and the NAS report on saccharin (1978).

Lessons Learned

In spite of the numerous toxicologic studies on this chemical, its true toxicity remains uncertain. The saccharin episode clearly indicates that:

1. Requirements for toxicologic data have been increasing in recent years.
2. More information was required following its greatly expanded use.
3. Many unforeseen complicating factors were encountered in most of these tests.
4. The need for reporting experimental details can be clearly seen.

GUIDELINES ON TESTING PROCEDURES: GENERAL ASPECTS

In designing a toxicologic test, consideration should be given to a number of factors that can influence the experimental results. The major ones follow.

Physicochemical Characteristics

Information on the purity and stability of the chemical to be tested is essential. The *impurities* in some chemicals are much more toxic than the chemicals themselves. For example, the herbicide 2,4,5-trichlorophenoxyacetic acid (2,4,5-T) has been found to contain an impurity, 2,3,7,8-tetrachlorodibenzo-dioxin (TCDD), which is much more toxic than 2,4,5-T. There are advantages in testing a chemical in its pure form, and there are advantages in testing the "technical grade," especially if it is relatively consistent from one batch to another with respect to the nature and quantity of the impurities.

Some chemicals degrade on *storage*. The degradation products can be more toxic or less so. In testing chemicals that are unstable, freshly prepared material must be used.

In some instances, a change in the *manufacturing process* of a chemical can alter its toxicity. For example, a brand of sulfaphenazole had been on the market for several years without any serious side effects. However, when a new manufacturing process was introduced, the drug caused convulsions in some young children and lowered the threshold to electric shock in rats. The effect in the rat was shown to be due to the impurities (Rice et al., 1965).

Other physicochemical properties of a chemical such as the pH, solubility in water and other solvents, and particle size as well as the vehicle, if used, can influence the local effects and the rate and extent of absorption, which can in turn modify the toxic manifestations.

Biologic Variables

The *species* and *strain* of the animals used in a toxicologic study must be recorded, since other species and strains may respond to a toxicant differently. When available information indicates that the biotransformation of a chemical is similar in humans and in a particular species or strain of animal, then these animals should be used, wherever feasible.

Unless otherwise indicated, testing for toxicity should be done in both sexes. If young children are likely to be particularly exposed and where information on biotransformation so indicates, the acute toxicity tests should be conducted on preweaning animals and/or neonates.

In general, the animals on tests are given feed and water *ad libitum*. Where the palatability of a chemical adversely affects the feed consumption and the body and organ weights, it may be useful to institute "paired feeding" to differentiate the effects of undernutrition from the true toxic effect of the chemical. Furthermore, the feed and water should be free from toxicologically significant toxic substances (e.g., aflatoxins) and enzyme inducers (e.g., DDT).

Other Factors

It is well known that the *duration* of exposure can alter the manifestation of toxicity of a chemical. Further, as a rule, increasing *doses* will increase the frequency of the response and they can even elicit different toxic effects. Such dose-response and dose-effect relationships can be well illustrated with the epidemiologic findings on methyl mercury (see Fig. 6-1) as well as with studies in animals.

At least one of the *routes* of administration of the chemicals to the animals should simulate the expected human exposure.

It is also well known that many of the effects of toxicants are seen in *control* animals. The toxicants may either increase their incidence or accelerate their appearance. It is, therefore, necessary to include a group of control animals that are subjected to the same experimental conditions (including such processes as sham operation, administration of the vehicle alone) as the treated animals, except that they are not exposed to the chemical on test. The importance of "historical" controls, in addition to "concurrent" controls, has been reviewed and emphasized (Task Force, 1982). Under certain conditions it is advisable to include a "positive control" group to ensure that the test animals have the expected response to a chemical possessing a known toxic effect, such as carcinogenicity.

Some of the effects can be readily quantified, e.g., mortality, body weight, and organ weight. Quantitative data are more amenable to *statistical analysis*. On the other hand, morphologic changes are often subject to individual judgment. Various procedures are being devised to quantify such changes.

Furthermore, a sufficient *number* of animals should be included in a toxicologic test. This will reduce the influence of variation in individual susceptibility. An even larger number of animals is required for tests in which the expected effect of a toxicant occurs spontaneously in control animals. For example, when groups of 50 animals are used, an effect that has an incidence of 8% can be detected (at a probability level of 0.025), provided that the effect does not occur in the controls. If the effect has a spontaneous incidence of 10%, then the toxicant in question will have to induce that effect in 26% of the treated animals to be considered significant.

Protocols Versus Guidelines

The generally held view among toxicologists is that toxicologic testing procedures should be flexible in order to permit full range exploration of the toxic effects of chemicals on tests. For example, the Joint FAO/WHO Expert Committee on Food Additives states in its Second Report (WHO, 1957): "No single pattern of tests could cover adequately, but not wastefully, the testing of substances so diverse in structure as food additives. . . . For this reason, the Committee concluded that it was only possible to formulate general recommendations with regard to testing procedure." The committee has adhered to this principle at all its subsequent annual meetings.

However, rigid protocols have been formulated by certain national regulatory authorities and routinely used in industry. Such protocols simplify the task of those in charge of testing and are designed to provide specific answers frequently required by industry and national regulatory agencies.

One must bear in mind that experimental results from some testing may indicate that additional studies ought to be undertaken even if these are not included in the protocol. Furthermore, advances in toxicology and allied sciences will necessitate periodic review and revision of the protocol. Nevertheless, a protocol designed for a specific study is useful in the proper planning and management of toxicity testing programs. The characteristics of several working protocols compiled by Gralla (1981b) is reproduced as Table 6-2.

GOOD LABORATORY PRACTICE

In 1975 and 1976, the U.S. Food and Drug Administration (FDA) raised questions about the integrity of toxicologic data received from certain laboratories. On inspecting these facilities, FDA discovered a number of unacceptable laboratory practices, such as selective reporting, underreporting, lack of adherence to a specified protocol, poor animal care procedures, poor recordkeeping, and inadequate supervision of personnel. In an attempt to improve the validity of the data, FDA proposed a set of regulations for good laboratory practice in 1978. These are later included in the Regulation for the Enforcement of the Federal Food, Drug, and Cosmetic Act.

These regulations (FDA, 1980) contain detailed guidance on provisions for the following:

1 Personnel, stipulating the responsibilities of the study director, testing facility management, and quality assurance unit
2 Facilities for animal care, animal supply, and handling test and control chemicals
3 Equipment, regarding its design, maintenance, and calibration
4 Testing facilities operation, including standard operating procedures, reagents and solutions, and animal care
5 Test and control chemicals, such as their characterization and handling
6 The protocol and conduct of a laboratory study
7 Records, its storage, retrieval and retention, as well as the preparation and contents of reports
8 Disqualifications of testing facilities

The U.S. Environmental Protection Agency also proposed a set of good laboratory practice standards. They contain provisions similar to those of the FDA regulation regarding health effects testing. However, the EPA standards also contain provisions for environmental effects testing (EPA, 1979).

A book edited by Gralla (1981a) includes useful pointers on a variety of topics, such as protocol preparation, quality assurance for rodents, quality

Table 6-2 Design Characteristics of Working Protocols[*] Used in the Study of Chemical Safety Evaluation

Purpose	Source	Length	Other features
Preclinical toxicology drug candidates	Food and Drug Administration or Pharmaceutical Manufacturing Association Guidelines	Single dose to 18 mo of daily dosing	• Three or more dose levels • Two, sometimes three, species • Expected clinical usage determines route and length of dosing • Complete laboratory work-up • Terminal sacrifice • Examine all animals for pathology
Preclinical toxicology of anticancer drug candidates	National Cancer Institute, Laboratory of Toxicology, Division of Cancer Treatment	Single dose to 10 wk	• All of the above • Pairs of animals on each dose level • Variable and interrupted treatment schedule • Includes nontreatment recovery periods
Bioassay for carcinogenicity	National Cancer Institute, Division of Cancer Cause and prevention	Two years in rodents (rats and mice)	• Two fixed feed levels • Examine all animals for pathology • Terminal nontreatment period
Bioassay for carcinogenicity	Food and Drug Administration, Bureau of Foods	Three generations	• Three dose levels • *In utero* exposure • Partial pathology and histopathology
Examine for toxicity and carcinogenicity	Chemical Industry Institute of Toxicology	Lifetime in rodents	• Dosed as mg/kg/day • Clinical laboratory • Interim sacrifices • Routine pathology on high dose and controls

Source: Gralla, 1981a.

[*]Defined as being available as a detailed written document and having been followed in the conduct of published studies.

assurance in clinical laboratory and in pathology, spontaneous lesions in rats and mice, and data collection, recordkeeping, and reporting results.

Adherence to good laboratory practice will improve the reliability of toxicologic data. It may also enhance international acceptance of such data, as pointed out by van Raalte (1980).

REFERENCES

Atallah, Y. H., and Whitacre, D. M. (1980) Industrial chemical safety testing: One company's approach. *Ecotoxicol. Environ. Safety* 4:357–361.

Bakir, F., Damluji, S., Amin-Zaki, L., Murtadha, M., Khalidi, A., Al-Rawi, N., Tikriti, S., Dhahir, H., Clarkson, T., Smith, J., and Doherty, R. (1973) Methylmercury poisoning in Iraq. An interuniversity report. *Science* 181: 230–241.

EPA (1979) Proposed health effects test standards for Toxic Substance Control Act test rules. *Federal Register* 44(91):27362–27369.

FDA (1980) Good laboratory practice for non-clinical laboratory studies. *Code of Federal Regulations*. Title 21, Part 58. Washington, D.C.: U.S. Government Printing Office.

Food Safety Council (1980) *Proposed System for Food Safety Assessment.* Washington, D.C.: Food Safety Council.

Gralla, E. J., ed. (1981a) *Scientific Consideration in Monitoring and Evaluating Toxicological Research.* Washington, D.C.: Hemisphere.

Gralla, E. J. (1981b) Protocol preparation: Design and objectives. In: *Scientific Consideration in Monitoring and Evaluating Toxicological Research.* Ed. E. J. Gralla. Washington, D.C.: Hemisphere.

International Agency on Research on Cancer (IARC) (1980) *Some Non-Nutritive Sweeteners.* IARC Monographs, Vol. 22. Lyon, France: International Agency on Research on Cancer.

National Academy of Sciences (1965) *Some Consideration in the Use of Human Subjects in Safety Evaluation of Pesticides and Food Chemicals.* NAS–NRC Publication 1270. Washington, D.C.: National Academy of Sciences.

National Academy of Sciences (1978) *Saccharin: Technical Assessment of Risks and Benefits.* Washington, D.C.: National Academy of Sciences.

Price, J. M., Biava, C. G., Oser, B. L., Vogin, E. E., Steinfeld, J., and Ley, H. L. (1970) Bladder tumors in rats fed cyclohexylamine or high doses of a mixture of cyclamate and saccharin. *Science* 167:1131–1132.

van Raalte, H. G. S. (1980) Acceptability of data from other countries. *Ecotoxicol. Environ. Safety* 4:466–467.

Rice, W. B., Lu, F. C., and Allmark, M. G. (1965) Stimulant effects of a sulfonamide preparation, sulfaphenazole, on the central nervous system in rats. *Can. Med. Assoc. J.* 92:180–181.

Task Force (1982) Animal data in hazard evaluation: Paths and pitfalls. Task Force of Past Presidents of the Society of Toxicology. *Fundam. Appl. Toxicol.* 2:101–107.

WHO (1957) *Procedures for the Testing of Intentional Food Additives to Establish Their Safety for Use.* WHO Tech. Rep. Ser. No. 144.

WHO (1976) *Environmental Health Criteria 1, Mercury.* Geneva: World Health Organization.

WHO (1978) Some general aspects of toxicity evaluation. In: *Environmental Health Criteria 6.* Geneva: World Health Organization.

Chapter 7

Toxicologic Evaluation

GENERAL CONSIDERATIONS

Toxicologic evaluation involves first a determination of the toxicity of the chemical, usually in a variety of biologic systems and under different exposure conditions. Second, an estimation is made of the safety/risk entailed in a specified exposure to the chemical in humans. Whereas the toxicity of a chemical is its inherent capacity to cause injury to a living organism, injury may not result from an exposure to the chemical if its amount is sufficiently small. However, the many experimental limitations and modifying factors involved in the toxicologic evaluation make it impossible to determine precisely the absolutely safe exposure. Thus the generally accepted definition of safety is the practical certainty that injury will not result from the chemical when used in the quantity and in the manner proposed for its use. The expression "practical certainty" can be defined either in terms of a numerically specified low risk or in terms of socially acceptable risks. Risk denotes the probability (expected frequency) that a chemical will produce undesirable effect under specified conditions.

The toxicity of a chemical is determined on the basis of sufficient relevant data, a numbeer of general aspects of which care included in Chapter 6. The safety/risk of the chemical, under a specified exposure condition, can be estimated using the toxicity data plus the data concerning the effects of various modifying factors. In addition, it is customary to use an appropriate safety factor or a mathematical model. The use of a factor or a model is intended to allow, on the basis of scientific knowledge and judgment, an extrapolation of the toxicity data from responses in animals given relatively large doses to the expected responses with exposures to small doses in humans. It is also intended to cover the differences in susceptibility between animals and humans, as well as a number of other uncertainties.

EXTRAPOLATION

From Animals to Humans

In general, humans are qualitatively similar to other animals in response to toxicants, except for those effects that are unique to humans, e.g., headache, loss of libido (Litchfield, 1961). This fact forms the basis of extrapolating data from animals to humans. However, there are quantitative differences between species. As a rule, humans are more susceptible than animals, especially when the dose is expressed in terms of mg/kg of body weight. While this is not invariably true [e.g., penicillin is lethal to guinea pigs and so is fluroxene to dogs, cats, and rabbits (Wardell, 1973)], for the sake of prudence, humans are considered more sensitive in the absence of any data to the contrary.

From Large Dose to Small Dose

In toxicologic studies, the doses selected are usually larger than those that are encountered by humans. This practice is followed because according to the principles of dose-effect and dose-response relationships, larger doses are expected to facilitate the identification of target organs and to reduce the need of using very large numbers of animals. Extrapolation of the observed dose-response relationship to an expected response at much lower doses requires critical consideration of other relevant data. For example, a large dose may overload various detoxication mechanisms of the host so that the effect observed may not occur with a small dose. The "carcinogenic" effect of Myrj 45 (see "Carcinogenic Chemicals") is observable only when the dose is large enough to produce bladder calculi, and the liver toxicity of furosemide is induced only after a large dose, which raised the level in the liver much more in relation to the increase of the dose.

From a Small Number to a Large Number of Organisms

Individual variations, as discussed in Chapter 5, exist in all species of animals. Human populations are much more heterogeneous than laboratory animals and thus are more variable in susceptibility to toxicants. Consequently, in extrapolating from a limited animal data base to the expected human responses, a safety factor is often used to compensate for the differences in individual variations between a small number of animals and a large human population. With mathematical models, as will be noted later in this chapter, a safety factor is included by the use of the upper confidence limits of the toxicity data, instead of the data themselves, or other procedures.

ACCEPTABLE DAILY INTAKE

Definition and Usage

The term *acceptable daily intake* (ADI) was coined by the Joint FAO/WHO Expert Committee on Food Additives in 1961 (WHO, 1962a). It has been adopted by the Joint FAO/WHO Meeting of Experts on Pesticide Residues (WHO, 1962b). This term has been used at all subsequent meetings of these two international expert bodies in their toxicologic evaluation, and re-evaluation, of large numbers of food additives and pesticides that leave residues in food.

ADI is defined as "the daily intake of a chemical which, during an entire lifetime, appears to be without appreciable risk on the basis of all the known facts at the time. It is expressed in milligrams of the chemical per kilogram of body weight (mg/kg)." It is worth noting that the ADI is qualified by the expressions "appear to be," and "on the basis of all the known facts at the time." This caution is in keeping with the fact that it is impossible to be absolutely certain about the safety of a chemical and that the ADI may be altered in the light of new toxicologic data.

Toxicologic evaluations of food additives and pesticides, in terms of ADIs by these international expert bodies, have been used by the regulatory agencies in many countries as an important consideration in the formulation of national regulations. ADIs have also been used collectively by national authorities in the framework of the Codex Alimentarius Commission. The Commission is an intergovernmental body with about 120 countries as members. Its principal function is to elaborate international food standards for the protection of the health of the consumer and to facilitate international food trade. These food standards contain provisions for food additives that are accepted by the Commission only when ADIs have been allocated by the Expert Committee on Food Additives.

Furthermore, the ADI is used as a yardstick to check the acceptability of the proposed uses. This is done by comparing the ADI with the "potential" daily intake, which is the sum of the amounts of the additive in each food calculated on the basis of the average per capita consumption of the foods and the permitted use levels in them. If the potential daily intake exceeds the ADI, the use levels may be lowered or some of the uses may be deleted. The Commission follows the same procedure in accepting the maximum limits for pesticide residues in food.

Additional details about the Codex Alimentarius Commission and the use of ADIs and potential daily intakes are given in two articles by Lu (1968, 1973).

Procedure for Estimating ADIs

Determination of the No-Effect Level The first step in estimating an ADI of a chemical is to assess whether the available data are sufficient to define the toxicologic profile of the substance involved. If they are, a no-effect level (NEL) is determined. This is the maximum dose level that has not induced any sign of toxicity in the most susceptible species of animals tested and using the most sensitive indicator of toxicity. As a rule, this level is selected from a long-term study. However, certain signs of toxicity, e.g., cataract, delayed neurotixicity, are demonstrable in short-term studies. The NEL is not necessarily an absolutely no-effect level; rather it is a "no *observed* effect level," because the use of a more sensitive indicator of toxicity or a more susceptible animal species may reveal a lower NEL. In addition, an effect might well be demonstrable if a sufficiently large number of animals were used in the test. However, the general consensus is that there is an absolute NEL no matter how large the dose groups are.

On the other hand, certain effects are generally considered as physiologic, adaptive, or otherwise "nontoxic." These effects are therefore excluded in establishing the NEL. For example, liver enlargement may result from stimulation in the activity of hepatic mixed-function oxidases and in the de novo protein synthesis in the smooth endoplasmic reticulum. A decrease of body weight may follow reduced food consumption, which in turn may be a result of unpalatability of the chemical. A reduction in liver glycogen or alteration in leukocyte count may not be indicative of a toxic effect but an adaptation to a stress situation. However, before disregarding these effects in evaluating the toxicity of a chemical, care must be taken to ensure that these are not manifestations of toxicity. Additional studies may have to be done to elucidate the nature of the effect. These various points have been elaborated in several WHO Reports (e.g., WHO, 1967; 1974a).

Safety Factors To extrapolate from the NEL in animals to an acceptable intake in humans, a safety factor of 100, originally proposed by Lehman and Fitzhugh (1954), is generally used. This factor is intended to allow for differences in sensitivity of the animal species and humans, to allow for wide variations in susceptibility among the human population, and to allow for the fact that the number of animals tested is small compared to the size of the human population that may be exposed (WHO, 1958, 1974a; NAS, 1970).

While the factor 100 is often used, the WHO expert committees have used figures that ranged from 10–2000. The size of the safety factor is determined according to the nature of the toxicity. In addition, a larger figure is used to compensate for slight deficiencies of toxicity data, e.g., small numbers of animals on test. On the other hand, available human data may warrant the use of a smaller figure since they obviate the need for interspecies extrapolation.

Biochemical data relating to the absorption, distribution, and excretion of the toxicant and its biotransformation (detoxication and bioactivation) in various species of animals and in humans are often useful in determining the size of the safety factor. These and other bases for altering the safety factor are elaborated in two WHO documents (WHO, 1967; 1974a).

MATHEMATICAL MODELS

Uniqueness of Carcinogenicity

Carcinogenicity is generally considered unique for several reasons. First, cancer cells can be induced by a single change in the cellular genetic material and second, they are self-replicating. Therefore, theoretically, a single molecule of a chemical can induce a cancer. In other words, there would be no threshold dose for carcinogens.

This view, however, is not universally accepted, because of the existence in the body of mechanisms that can prevent the initiation and progression of carcinogenesis. Among these are detoxication and excretion of the toxicant, its covalent binding with noncritical macromolecules, DNA repair, immunologic surveillance, and protective agents, such as antioxidants. Although these mechanisms would increase the minimal amount of a carcinogen to induce cancer, the existence of threshold doses for carcinogenic chemicals has not been satisfactorily demonstrated, not even with the largest experiment (over 24,000 mice) carried out on 2-acetylaminofluorene (Littlefield et al., 1979; SOT ED_{01} Task Force, 1981).

In the absence of a reliable procedure to determine a threshold for a carcinogen for an entire population (WHO, 1974b; IRLG, 1979; OSHA, 1980), estimating the levels of risk has been considered to be more appropriate.

Estimation of Risks

Definition   Risk has been defined as the expected frequency of undesirable effects arising from exposure to a pollutant. It may be expressed in absolute terms as the risk due to exposure to a specific pollutant. It may also be expressed as a relative risk, which is the ratio of the risk among the exposed population to that among the unexposed (WHO, 1978).

The term was first adopted by the International Commission on Radiological Protection (ICRP, 1966) in evaluating the health hazards related to ionizing radiation. The use of this term stems from the realization that often a clear-cut "safe" or "unsafe" decision cannot be made.

Risks Levels and Virtual Safety Estimation of risks involves development of suitable dose-response data and extrapolation from the observed dose-response relationship to the expected responses at doses occurring at actual exposure situations. A number of mathematical models have been proposed in recent years for this purpose. Such models are also used to estimate the dose that is expected to be associated with a specific level of risk.

Mantel and Bryan (1961) first introduced the concept of virtual safety. The term was defined as a probability of carcinogenicity of less than 1/100 million (10^{-8}) at a statistical assurance level of 99%. The U.S. Food and Drug Administration, however, found that the doses associated with such a low risk level were too small to be enforceable in most actual situations and thus adopted a risk level of 10^{-6} (FDA, 1977). These levels of risk are so low that the doses associated with them are referred to as virtual safe doses (VSD).

Commonplace Activities and Their Risks In order to place the risk levels in perspective, risks associated with certain commonplace activities and natural occurrences are sometimes cited. Table 7-1 includes a number of estimates of such risks.

The risks in Table 7-1, apart from lightning, are considerably greater than 10^{-6}. Estimates of risks associated with other common activities and occupations have been compiled by others, for example, Wilson (1980).

The acceptability of a risk depends on, apart from its magnitude, the nature of the activity. In general, risks associated with voluntary, pleasurable, and/or beneficial activities, such as smoking and driving, are more acceptable to the individual. On the other hand, risks associated with activities that are perceived as having no benefit and those that are not controllable by the individual tend to be rejected, e.g., food additives suspected of being carcinogenic. A number of

Table 7-1   Estimated Risks for Certain Activities and Natural Occurrences

Activity	Risk[*]
Smoking (10 cigarettes/day)	1/400
All accidents	1/2,000
Driving (16,000 km/year)	1/5,000
All traffic accidents	1/8,000
Work in industry	1/30,000
Natural disasters	1/50,000
Being struck by lightning	1/1,000,000

Source: Adapted from Royal Commission on the Environment, 1976. By permission of the Controller of Her Majesty's Stationery Office, London.

[*]Risk is expressed as probability of death of an individual for a year of exposure and is given in round figures.

other factors can also affect the acceptability of various categories of risks as pointed out by the Science Council of Canada (1977).

Models for Estimating VSD

Conservative Models A number of models have been developed for this purpose. They involve, in general, extrapolating from the observed dose-response to the VSD on the basis of certain assumptions about the mathematical nature of the dose-response relationship near zero dose. These models yield widely different VSDs. The FDA Panel on Carcinogenesis (1971) calculated the VSDs at 10^{-6} and 10^{-8} with the probit, logistic, and one-particle models. The VSDs expressed as fractions of the median tumor dose (TD_{50}) are shown in the following:

Risk Level	Probit	Logistic	One-Particle
10^{-6}	1.36×10^{-3}	9.8×10^{-6}	1.44×10^{-6}
10^{-8}	4.12×10^{-4}	1.6×10^{-7}	1.40×10^{-8}

Although there is a difference of 1000-fold at 10^{-6} and nearly 30,000-fold at 10^{-8} between the VSDs calculated with the probit and one-particle models, the relative merits of these models cannot be ascertained experimentally because the "observed" dose-responses fit these three models equally well, as shown by the Panel.

The conservativeness of these models is achieved through the use of upper confidence limits to responses, shallow slopes, or the lower confidence limits on the VSD estimated. Because of this conservativeness, the VSDs derived from these models tend to be very small. Such small VSDs are in most cases unenforceable and perhaps unnecessarily conservative. In recent years, less conservative models based on certain biologic reasons have therefore been developed, and these are referred to as stochastic models.

Stochastic Models The *multi-hit model* assumes that several hits are required for a response to occur. In contrast, the *one-hit model* assumes that one will suffice. The *multi-stage model* is built on the assumption that the induction of a carcinogenic response follows random biological events, the time rate of occurrence of each event being in linear proportion to the dose rate.

Other Variations *Linear extrapolation* has been endorsed by the U.S. Interagency Regulatory Liaison Group (IRLG, 1979). It involves essentially connecting, with a straight line, the origin (zero dose) and the upper confidence limit of the response at the lowest experimental dose and determining the VSD that corresponds to the desired risk level, using the straight line. Figure 7-1 shows the observed responses, the upper confidence limit, and the linear interpo-

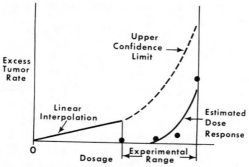

Figure 7-1 Linear extrapolation showing the observed responses, the upper confidence limit of the response at the lowest experimental dose, and the linear interpolation (from Gaylor and Kodell, 1980).

lation. The *Weibull Model* is a weighted least-square regression program. It has been endorsed by the Food Safety Council (1980). Further, a program written for an electronic calculator that handles up to nine data points to fit this model has been designed for the Council.

The time-to-response, instead of the response itself, has also been proposed for use in the mathematical models (Chand and Hoel, 1974; Sielken, 1981). The importance of this approach has been pointed out by the SOT ED_{01} Task Force (1981) and the Task Force (1982). Background responses, i.e., those occurring among the unexposed, are often observed. They can also be incorporated into mathematical models (Hoel, 1980; Van Ryzin and Rai, 1980).

The response of an organism to a toxicant is related to the dose and the duration of exposure. It is also affected by competing risks. Kalbfleisch et al. (1983) proposed mathematical models that will take these three factors into account.

Incorporation of *metabolism data* into mathematical models represents an important refinement. Since vinyl chloride is carcinogenic after bioactivation, Gehring et al. (1978) showed that the tumor incidence in rats exposed to various concentrations of this chemical was proportional to the metabolized amount rather than the exposure concentration. This conclusion is evident from the data summarized in Table 7-2.

Since many carcinogens require bioactivation, the importance of incorporating metabolic data in evaluating their risks is obvious. Furthermore, Anderson et al. (1980) suggest that the DNA-carcinogen adduct formed should be used instead of the amount of the parent compound or its reactive metabolite.

OTHER PROCEDURES

Noncarcinogenic Chemicals

Not all chemicals require the whole gamut of toxicologic testing as described for estimating ADIs. For example, for chemicals that humans are not likely to be exposed to an appreciable extent, such as indirect food additives and certain pesticides, a "toxicologically insignificant amount" may be estimated on the basis of toxicologic data that include at least 90-day feeding studies in two species of mammals and by the use of a larger safety factor (NAS, 1965; FDA, 1980).

Furthermore, a decision to reject a chemical may be made on much limited data, especially in the course of developing new chemicals. Such data include extreme acute toxicity, positive response in short-term mutagenesis tests, or undesirable features in biochemical studies or short-term feeding studies in animals (see Table 6-2).

Carcinogenic Chemicals

The Joint FAO/WHO Expert Committee on Food Additives as its second meeting (WHO, 1958) recommended that "no proved carcinogen should be considered suitable for use as a food additive in any amount." This principle has been followed at subsequent meetings of the Committee and at the Joint FAO/WHO Meetings on Pesticide Residues in not allocating ADIs to proved carcinogens. *Temporary or conditional ADIs*, however, have been estimated for chemicals with equivocal carcinogenicity data, e.g., nitrites and DDT. On the other hand, discontinuation of the use of chemicals without essential functions has been recommended. The basis for the decisions on these and other such chemicals have been reviewed and summarized (Lu, 1979). This principle of considering both the soundness of the carcinogenesis data and the usefulness of the chemical is consistent with the policies of many national regulatory agencies.

On the other hand, it has been proposed that for carcinogens with important uses, a *probable safe level* for humans can be estimated by applying a safety factor of 5000 to the minimum effective dose in well-conducted cancer experiments in animals (Weil, 1972; Truhaut, 1979).

The concept of *secondary carcinogens*, which induce tumor only after

Table 7-2 Correlation between Exposure Concentration of Vinyl Chloride (VC), Metabolism, and Induction of Hepatic Angiosarcoma in Rats

Exposure concentration (ppm of VC)	μg of VC/liter of air	μg of VC metabolized	Percentage liver angiosarcoma
50	128	739	2
250	640	2,435	7
500	1,280	3,413	12
2,500	6,400	5,030	22
6,000	15,360	5,003	22
10,000	25,600	5,521	15

Source: Adapted from Gehring et al., 1978.

certain noncarcinogenic effect, has been accepted by many toxicologists. For example, a WHO scientific group (WHO, 1974b) pointed out that the urinary bladder cancers in rats treated with Myrj 45 (polyoxyethylene monostearate) were caused by the bladder calculi rather than the chemical directly and that a NEL can therefore be established. A variety of other types of secondary carcinogens have been enumerated by Golberg (1978).

In studies on the *mechanism of action*, Ramsey and Gehring (1980) showed that perchloroethylene (Perc) and vinylidene chloride (VDC), increased DNA synthesis only when there was tissue damage, in contrast to dimethylnitrosamine, which caused marked DNA damage and DNA repair. Furthermore, they noted that Perc and VDC do not induce tumors and do not increase DNA synthesis in rats. The authors therefore suggested that the predominant mechanism whereby a chemical elicits a carcinogenic response should be considered in extrapolating laboratory data to humans.

It is becoming more widely recognized that there are marked differences in the nature and extent of positive data among carcinogenic chemicals. Some chemicals, such as aflatoxin, consistently yield positive response in a variety of animals, with small doses and after a relatively short latent period, whereas others, such as saccharin, yield positive response inconsistently, and only with large doses and after long durations of treatment. These chemicals also differ in their mechanism of action and a number of other aspects. That these differences should be used in setting priorities in regulating carcinogens has been suggested by Kolbye (1976).

More recently, Munro and Krewski (1981) proposed that carcinogens should be classified according to a number of criteria: (1) number of species and strains affected, (2) number of tissue sites at which tumors occur, (3) latency period, (4) strength of dose required to induce tumors, (5) proportions of benign and malignant lesions, (6) nature and degree of other pathologic changes, (7) chemical similarity to other known carcinogens, (8) metabolic and pharmacokinetic data, (9) biochemical reactivity with DNA, RNA, and protein, and (10) genotoxicity and activity in short-term tests for carcinogenicity.

Squire (1981) devised a ranking system to evaluate carcinogens. Such chemicals are scored according to the following criteria: (1) number of species affected, (2) number of histogenetically different types of neoplasms in one or more species, (3) spontaneous incidence in appropriate control groups of neoplasms induced in treated groups, (4) dose-response relationships (cumulative oral dose equivalents per kilogram of body weight per day for 2 years), (5) malignancy of induced neoplasms, and (6) genotoxicity, measured in an appropriate battery of tests. Using the total score for each carcinogen, the author ranked, for example, aflatoxin as I; 2-naphthylamine, II; chloroform, III; NTA (nitrilotriacetic acid), IV; and saccharin, V. The value of this system in ranking carcinogens when the epidemiologic data are inadequate has been underlined by the Task Force of the Past Presidents of the Society of Toxicology (Task Force, 1982).

COMMENTS ON TWO WIDELY USED PROCEDURES

Acceptable Daily Intake

The widely adopted procedure for evaluating noncarcinogenic chemicals is to estimate their ADIs, based on the belief that there are threshold doses below which no adverse effects are expected from exposure to them. As noted above, many food additives, pesticides, and other chemicals have been so evaluated. This procedure has not excessively restricted the use of these chemicals and has failed only very rarely.

One such failure related to the myocardial effects observed among heavy drinkers of beer that contained 1 ppm cobalt. Cobalt chloride was added to beer as a foam stabilizer and to prevent gushing. Cobalt salts have long been used in the treatment of anemia at doses of about 300 mg/day. No heart lesions have been reported from such treatment. The heavy beer drinkers drank about 10 liters a day, containing therefore only one-thirtieth of the therapeutic dose of cobalt. Subsequent studies showed that the toxicity of cobalt was greatly enhanced by the malnutrition, especially the deficiency of certain amino acid, associated with a large caloric intake from the beer alone (Wiberg et al., 1969). The magnitude of potentiating effects of alcohol and malnutrition was not expected and therefore not taken into account in assessing the safety of cobalt in beer.

Another glaring failure in toxicologic evaluation resulted in the tragedy following the clinical use of thalidomide. This sedative/hypnotic was tested according to the then prevailing protocol and found to have a low toxicity. However, after its use in pregnant women, there appeared many cases of phocomelia from mothers who had taken this drug (Lenz and Knapp, 1962). This failure resulted, obviously, from a lack of appropriate prior testing for teratogenicity.

These two examples illustrate that toxicologic evaluations can be invalidated when there are significant, unexpected toxic effects or undetected but marked influences of modifying factors. They do not, however, signify an absence of threshold doses. Furthermore, the deficiency of biologic data cannot be overcome by mathematical manipulations of the available dose-response data.

Since it is impossible to be certain that all appropriate tests have been conducted on a chemical, a caveat must be included in any toxicologic evaluation. Apart from rigorous testing and cautious evaluation prior to the introduction of a new chemical to the human environment, it is prudent to monitor the exposed population for possible deleterious effects and to reassess its toxicologic implications in the light of new data and of improvements in toxicologic methodology (WHO, 1957).

Mathematical Models

These models have been used mainly in evaluating carcinogens, but they have also been proposed for use with noncarcinogens. This proposal was made because an absolute NEL cannot be determined in view of the limitations on the number of animals that can be used (Cornfield et al., 1978) and because the slope of the dose-response curve is not taken into account in the selection of a safety factor (Cornfield et al., 1980). Contrary to these views, it should be noted that the two points mentioned above are in fact considered by some toxicologists in deciding on the size of the safety factor, although only done according to "scientific judgment" rather than on a strict statistical basis.

Mathematical models have been used by the Food Safety Council (1980) in estimating the VSD with respect to the lethal effect of botulinum toxin. This seems to ignore the fundamental difference between carcinogens and noncarcinogens. The effect of the former is not only irreversible but also capable of self-replicating, whereas the latter is not. In other words, a critical hit by a carcinogen theoretically can induce a cancer, but botulinum toxin cannot act in this way. For this toxin to cause death, a huge number of myofibrils in the respiratory muscles must be paralyzed. Therefore, a dose that is too small to bind with a sufficient number of the receptors on the neurofibrils supplying these muscles cannot cause death, no matter how sensitive an individual is.

Furthermore, even with a toxicant, such as methyl mercury, that is capable of causing irreversible damages, a minimum dose is required to destroy a sufficient number of the 10^{11} neurons in the human brain to induce manifestations of the typical CNS symptoms and signs. Whereas the risk of having one or a few neurons irreversibly damaged by methyl mercury is always present with any dose of this toxicant, such damages are evidently of no health concern.

Even in considering risks of carcinogens, the mathematical models can only be considered as interim procedures. This is because, as pointed out by Munro and Krewski (1981), "animal studies serve primarily as qualitative surrogates for humans, and any attempts to quantify response beyond the realm of biological certainty are open to question."

The above view was also lucidly stated by the Task Force (1982) of Past Presidents of the Society of Toxicology, who quoted M. J. Winrow: "We have some extremely sophisticated, precise mathematical methods that are being applied to biological data, but however carefully the data are collected, they are going to vary because the biological part of the system varies." It is too easy ". . . to become mesmerized by the strings of precise numbers being churned out by computers, and to forget that the biological data going in aren't anywhere near so precise."

It is also worth noting that the estimated VSDs for the same chemical often differ by a factor of several orders of magnitude. This fact was illustrated by the FDA Panel on Carcinogenesis (1971) (see "Conservative Models") and is also evident among VSDs compiled by the Food Safety Council (1980). An extreme example is provided by the calculations on saccharin. The National Academy of Sciences (NAS, 1979) estimated the expected number of cases of bladder cancer in the United States due to lifetime exposure to 120 mg saccharin per day to range from 0.001–5200 cases per million individuals, a difference of 5.2 million-fold! Estimated VSDs with these models appear to be improved by incorporating relevant metabolic and pharmacokinetic data as shown with vinyl chloride (Table 7-2). It is hoped that the value of the models might be improved if they can be modified to take into account the other relevant biologic properties enumerated by Munro and Krewski (1981) and Squire (1981).

REFERENCES

Anderson, M. W., Hoel, D. G., and Kaplan, N. L. (1980) A general scheme for incorporation of pharmacokinetics in low-dose risk estimation for chemical carcinogenesis: Example–vinyl chloride. *Toxicol. Appl. Pharmacol.* 155: 154–161.

Chand, N., and Hoel, W. (1974) A comparison of models for determining safe levels of environmental agents. In: *Reliability and Biometry*, p. 681. Eds. F. Proschan and R. J Serfling, Philadelphia: SIAM.

Cornfield, J., Carlborg, P. N., and Van Ryzin, J. (1978) Setting tolerances on the basis of mathematical treatment of dose-response data extrapolated to low doses. In: *Proceedings of the First International Congress on Toxicology*, p. 143. Eds. G. L. Plaa and W. A. M. Duncan. New York: Academic Press.

Cornfield, J., Rai, K., and Van Ryzin, J. (1980) Procedures for assessing risk at low levels of exposure. *Arch. Toxicol.* 3(Suppl.):295.

FDA (1971) Food and Drug Administration Advisory Committee on Protocols for Safety Evaluation: Panel on Carcinogenesis report on cancer testing in the safety evaluation of food additives and pesticides. *Toxicol. Appl. Pharmacol.* 20:419–438.

FDA (1977) Chemical compounds in food-producing animals: Criteria and procedures for evaluating assays for carcinogenic residues in edible products of animals. *Fed. Regist.* 42(35):10412–10437.

FDA (1980) *Code of Federal Regulations.* Title 40, Section 181.1(1).

Food Safety Council (1980) Proposed System for Food Safety Assessment. *Food Cosmet. Toxicol.* 16, Suppl. 2.

Gaylor, D. W., and Kodell, R. L. (1980) Linear interpolation algorithm for low dose risk assessment of toxic substances. *J. Environ. Pathol. Toxicol.* 4: 305–312.

Gehring, P. J., Watanabe, P. G., and Park, C. N. (1978) Resolution of dose-response toxicity for chemicals requiring metabolic activation: Example–vinyl chloride. *Toxicol. Appl. Pharmacol.* 44:581–591.

Goldberg, L. (1978) Introductory remarks: Consideration of experimental thresholds. In: *Proceedings of the First International Congress on Toxicology*, pp. 87–95. Eds. G. L. Plaa and W. A. M. Duncan. New York: Academic Press.

Hoel, D. G. (1980) Incorporation of background in dose-response models. *Fed. Proc.* 39:73–75.

ICRP (1966) *Recommendations of the International Commission on Radiological Protection.* ICRP Publication No. 9. Oxford: Pergamon Press.

Interagency Regulatory Liaison Group (IRLG) (1979) The scientific basis for identification of potential carcinogens and risk estimation. *J. Nat. Cancer Inst.* 63:241–268; *Fed. Regist.* 44(131):39858–39879.

Kalbfleisch, J. D., Krewski, D., and van Ryzin, J. (1983) Dose-response models for time to response toxicity data. *Can. J. Stat.* 11:25–49.

Kolbye, A. C., Jr. (1976) Cancer in humans: Exposures and responses in a real world. *Oncology* 33:90–100.

Lehman, A. J., and Fitzhugh, O. G. (1954) 100-fold margin of safety. *Quart. Bull. Assoc. Food Drug Officials U.S.*, pp. 33–35.

Lenz, W., and Knapp, K. (1962) Thalidomide embryopathy. *Arch. Environ. Health* 5:100–105.

Litchfield, J. T., Jr. (1961) Forecasting drug effects in man from studies in laboratory animals. *JAMA* 177:34–38.

Littlefield, N. A., Farmer, J. H., Gaylor, C. W., and Sheldon, W. G. (1979) Effects of dose and time in long-term, low-dose carcinogenic study. *J. Environ. Pathol. Toxicol.* 3:17–34.

Lu, F. C. (1968) The Joint FAO/WHO Food Standards Program and the Codex Alimentarious. *WHO Chron.* 24:198–205.

Lu, F. C. (1973) Toxicological evaluation of food additives and pesticide residues and their "acceptable daily intakes" for man: The role of WHO, in conjunction with FAO. *Residue Rev.* 45:81–93.

Lu, F. C. (1979) Assessment at an international level of health hazards to man of chemicals shown to be carcinogenic in laboratory animals. In: *Regulatory Aspects of Carcinogenesis and Food Additives: The Delaney Clause.* Ed. F. Coulston. New York: Academic Press.

Mantel, N., and Bryan, W. R. (1961) "Safety" testing of carcinogenic agents. *J. Nat. Cancer Inst.* 27:455–470.

Munro, I. C., and Krewski, D. R. (1981) Risk assessment and regulatory decision making. *Food Cosmet. Toxicol.* 19:549–560.

National Academy of Sciences (NAS) (1965) *Report on "No Residue" and "Zero Tolerance."* Washington, D.C.: National Academy of Sciences.

National Academy of Sciences (NAS) (1970) *Evaluation the Safety of Food Chemicals.* Washington, D.C.: National Academy of Sciences.

National Academy of Sciences (NAS) (1979) *Saccharin: Technical Assessment of Risks and Benefits.* Washington, D.C.: National Academy of Sciences.

Occupational Safety and Health Administration (OSHA) (1980) Can "safe" or "no-effect" levels be set for exposure to carcinogens? *Federal Register* 45(15):5138.

Ramsey, J. C., and Gehring, P. J. (1980) Application of pharmacokinetic principles in practice. *Fed. Proc.* 39:60–65.

Royal Commission on the Environment (1976) *Sixth Report: Nuclear Power and the Environment.* London: Her Majesty's Stationery Office.

Science Council of Canada (1977) *Policies and Poisons: The Containment of Long-Term Hazards to Human Health in the Environment and in the Workplace.* Don Mills, Ontario: Thorn Press.

Sielken, R. L., Jr. (1981) Re-examination of the ED_{01} study: Risk assessment using time. *Funda. Appl. Toxicol.* 1:88–123.

SOT ED_{01} Task Force (1981) Re-examination of the ED_{01} Study. *Funda. Appl. Toxicol.* 1:26–128.

Squire, R. A. (1981) Ranking carcinogens: A proposed regulatory approach. *Science* 214:877-880.

Task Force (1982) Animal data in hazard evaluation: Paths and pitfalls. Task Force of Past Presidents of the Society of Toxicology. *Funda. Appl. Toxicol.* 2:101-107.

Truhaut, R. (1979) An overview of the problem of thresholds for chemical carcinogens. In: *Carcinogenic Risks/Strategies for Intervention.* Eds. W. Davis and E. Rosenfeld. IARC Scientific Publication No. 25, p. 191, Lyon, France: International Agency for Research on Cancer.

Van Ryzin, J., and Rai, K. (1980) The use of quantal data to make predictions. In: *The Scientific Basis of Toxicity Assessment.* Ed. H. R. Witschi. New York: Elsevier.

Wardell, W. M. (1972) Fluroxene and the penicillin lesson. *Anesthesiology* 38: 309-312.

Weil, C. S. (1972) Statistics vs. safety factors and scientific judgement in the evaluation of safety for man. *Toxicol. Appl. Pharmacol.* 21:454-463.

WHO (1957) *General Principles Governing the Use of Food Additives.* First Report of the Joint FAO/WHO Expert Committee on Food Additives. WHO Tech. Rep. Ser. No. 129.

WHO (1958) *Procedures for the Testing of Intentional Food Additives to Establish Their Safety in Use.* Second Report. WHO Tech. Rep. Ser. No. 144.

WHO (1962a) *Evaluation of the Toxicity of a Number of Antimicrobials and Antioxidants.* Sixth Report. WHO Tech. Rep. Ser. No. 228.

WHO (1962b) *Principles Governing Consumer Safety in Relation to Pesticide Residues.* Report of a Joint FAO/WHO Meeting on Pesticide Residues. WHO Tech. Rep. Ser. No. 240.

WHO (1967) *Procedures for Investigating Intentional and Unintentional Food Additives.* WHO Tech. Rep. Ser. No. 348.

WHO (1974a) *Toxicological Evaluation of Certain Food Additives with a Review of General Principles and of Specifications.* Seventeenth Report. WHO Tech. Rep. Ser. No. 539.

WHO (1974b) *Assessment of the Carcinogenicity and Mutagenicity of Chemicals.* Report of a WHO Scientific Group. WHO Tech. Rep. Ser. No. 546.

WHO (1978) *Principles and Methods for Evaluatiorg the Toxicity of Chemicals.* Environmental Health Criteria 6. Geneva: World Health Organization.

Wiberg, G. S., Munro, I. C., Meranger, J. C., Morrison, A. B., and Grice, H. C. (1969) Factors affecting the cardiotoxic potential of cobalt. *Clin. Toxicol.* 2:257-271.

Wilson, R. (1980) Risk/benefit analysis for toxic chemicals. *Ecotoxicol. Environ. Safety* 4:370-383.

ADDITIONAL READINGS

Corn, M. (1980) Regulatory toxicology. In: *Casarett and Doull's Toxicology.* Eds. J. Doull, C. D. Klaassen, and M. O. Amdur. New York: Macmillan.

Gaylor, D. W. (1980) The ED_{01} study: Summary and conclusions. *J. Environ. Pathol. Toxicol.* 3:179-183.

Part Two

Testing Procedures

Chapter 8

Acute, Short–Term, and Long–Term Toxicity Studies

GENERAL CONSIDERATIONS

The effects of toxicants are related *inter alia* to the duration of exposure. In order to examine the different effects associated with various lengths of exposure, toxicologic studies are generally divided into three categories: (1) *acute toxicity studies*, which involve either a single administration of the chemical under test or several administrations within a 24-hour period. (2) *Short-term* (also known as subacute and subchronic) toxicity studies, which involve repeated administrations, usually on a daily or 5 times per week basis, over a period of about 10% of the life-span, namely 3 months in rats and 1 or 2 years in dogs. However, shorter durations such as 14- and 28-day treatments have also been used by some investigators. (3) *Long-term* toxicity studies, which involve repeated administrations over a period of the entire life-span of the test animals or at least a major fraction of it, e.g., 18 months in mice, 24 months in rats, and 7–10 years in dogs and monkeys.

ACUTE TOXICITY STUDIES

Most of such studies are designed to determine the median lethal dose (LD_{50}) of the toxicant. The LD_{50} has been defined as "a statistically derived expression of a single dose of a material that can be expected to kill 50% of the animals." In addition, such studies can also indicate the probable target organ of the chemical and its specific toxic effect and provide guidance on the doses to be used in the more prolonged studies.

When the route of exposure is inhalation, the endpoint is then either the median lethal concentration (LC_{50}) with a given duration of exposure or the median lethal time (LT_{50}) with a given concentration of the chemical in the air.

Experimental Design

Selection of Species of Animal In general, the rat and mouse are selected for use in determining the LD_{50}. Their preference stems from the fact that they are economical, readily available, and easy to handle. Further, there are more toxicologic data on these species of animals, a fact that facilitates comparisons of toxicities of other chemicals.

In addition, a nonrodent species is desirable. This is true especially when the LD_{50} values in rats and mice are markedly different or when the pattern or rate of biotransformation in humans is known to be significantly different from rats and mice.

The LD_{50} determination should be done in animals of both sexes, and also in adult and young animals, because of their differences in susceptibility.

Route of Administration Generally, the toxicant should be administered by the route by which humans would be exposed. The oral route is most commonly used. When a chemical is to be administered orally, it should be given by gavage. Mixing a chemical in the diet has the disadvantage of imprecise dosage and generally reducing the toxicity of the chemical.

A vehicle is usually required in dissolving or suspending the toxicant to facilitate its administration. Even when the toxicant is a liquid it may need a diluent. The vehicle per se should have little or no toxic effect, and it should not react with the toxicant. Common vehicles are such solvents as water, saline, vegetable gums, and cellulose derivatives.

The volume of the toxicant in solution or suspension can affect the toxicity. Excessively large volumes of a liquid can cause untoward effects to the animal. On the other hand, if the volume is reduced the concentration will be higher, a fact that can increase the toxicity (Ferguson, 1962; Griffith, 1964). Therefore, when a large amount of a toxicant is to be administered to an animal, it may be advisable to give it in divided doses.

The dermal and inhalation routes are used increasingly, not only for chemicals that are intended for human use by such routes but also for chemicals whose health hazards to personnel handling these chemicals are to be assessed.

Parenteral routes are mainly used in assessing the acute toxicity of parenteral drugs. In addition, immediate or very prompt and complete or nearly complete absorption generally follow intravenous and intraperitoneal injection; these types of administration are also used to assess the rate and extent of absorption by the oral and dermal routes.

Dosage and Number of Animals The aim of the LD_{50} test is to determine the dose that would kill 50% of the animals and to determine the slope of the dose-response curve. It is therefore necessary to try to select a dose that would kill about half of the animals, another that would kill more than half (preferably less than 90%), and a third dose that would kill less than half (preferably more than 10%) of the animals. Four or more doses are often used in the hope that at least three of them would fall in the right range.

In general, the precision of the LD_{50} is improved by increasing the number of animals per dose and by decreasing the ratio between successive doses. Many investigators use about 50 animals per LD_{50} test and select ratios of 1.2–1.5. However, others (e.g., Weil, 1952) proposed the use of four animals per dose and a ratio of 2.0 between successive doses. According to his results (Weil et al., 1953), the LD_{50} values obtained with this simplified method are similar to those obtained with ten animals per dose and with a ratio of 1.26. However, the fiducial ranges are much wider. It is therefore obvious that for routine LD_{50} tests, the procedure proposed by Weil might be adequate.

On the other hand, there are occasions when a more precise determination of the LD_{50} is desired. A more precise LD_{50} can be obtained with a smaller ratio between successive doses. For example, a ratio of 1.2 has been used (Lu et al., 1965) in demonstrating a lack of appreciable diurnal variation and a marked difference in toxicity between batches. On the same batches of malathion, but using a ratio of 2 between successive doses, no conclusions could be drawn from the 100 LD_{50} determinations with respect to the differences between batches because of the wide confidence of limits (Shaffer, C. B., unpublished data).

A small ratio between successive doses is feasible only when information on its approximate acute toxicity is available. Otherwise, an approximate LD_{50} can be obtained by a preliminary test using a procedure such as that proposed by Weil (1952).

In determining the LD_{50} in large animals, e.g., dogs, generally a much smaller number of them are used.

Environmental Factors *Caging* can affect the LD_{50} of a chemical in several ways. For example, the LD_{50} of isoproterenol was less than 50 mg/kg in rats caged individually, whereas it was about 800 mg/kg in rats caged in groups of ten (Balazs, 1972). However, the LD_{50} values of most chemicals are only slightly affected, if at all, by this factor. The type of cage (mesh versus solid) and the type of litter material can also affect the reaction of the animals to toxicants.

Temperature of the environment can alter the toxic effect. For example, the toxicity of strychnine, nicotine, atropine, malathion, and sarin is increased in animals exposed to cold temperature. However, the toxicity of parathion, another organophosphorous insecticide, is reduced by hypothermia.

A higher relative *humidity* may increase the acute toxicity, resulting in a lower LD_{50} dose.

Because of the potential effect of these factors on the LD_{50}, the precise conditions under which the test is conducted should be noted and reported.

Observations and Examinations

After administering the toxicant to the animals, they should be examined not only for the number and time of death but also for central, autonomic, and behavior effects, including their onset, intensity, and duration. The frequency of these nonlethal effects should also be noted for each dosage group so that the LD_{50} dose for these effects might be estimated. Sperling (1976) discussed in detail the types of observations that should be made and the value of these observations. McNamara (1976) compiled a list of toxic signs and the systems and organs affected as a guide to facilitate the observations of the animals (Table 8-1).

The observation period should be sufficiently long so that delayed effects, including death, would not be missed. The period is usually 7–14 days but may be much longer.

Gross autopsies should be performed on all animals that have died as well as at least some of the survivors, especially those that are morbid at the termination of the experiment. Autopsy can provide useful information on the target organ, especially when death does not occur shortly after the dosing. Histopathologic examination of selected organs and tissues may also be indicated.

Evaluation of the Data

Dose-response Relationship Because of the variation of individual sensitivity of any group of organisms, they will not die of the same dose of a chemical. Therefore, the frequency of response, e.g., death, will increase along with the dose. When the mortality, or the frequency of other effects, is plotted against the dose on a logarithmic scale, an S-shaped curve is obtained. The central portion of the curve (between 16% and 84% response) is sufficiently straight for estimating the LD_{50} or ED_{50} dose. However, a much wider range of the curve can be straightened by plotting the points on a probit basis. This procedure is especially useful in estimating, for example, the LD_5 or ED_{95} dose, when the extreme ends of this curve have to be used.

The probit units correspond to normal equivalent deviations around the mean, e.g., $+1, +2, +3$ ... and $-1, -2, -3$ ... deviations, whereas the mean

Table 8-1 Relationship between Toxic Signs and Body Organs or Systems

System	Toxic signs
Autonomic	Relaxed nictitating membrane, exophthalmos, nasal discharge, salivation, diarrhea, urination, piloerection
Behavioral	Sedation, restlessness, sitting position-head up, staring straight ahead, drooping head, severe depression, excessive preening, gnawing paws, panting, irritability, aggressive and defensive hostility, fear, confusion, bizarre activity
Sensory	Sensitivity to pain; righting, corneal, labyrinth, placing, and hind limb reflex; sensitivity to sound and touch; nystagmus, phonation
Neuromuscular	Decreased and increased activity, fasciculation, tremors, convulsions, ataxia, prostration, straub tail, hind limb weakness, pain and hind limb reflexes (absent or diminished), opisthotonos, muscle tone, death
Cardiovascular	Increased and decreased heart rate, cyanosis, vasoconstriction, vasodilation, hemorrhage
Respiratory	Hypopnea, dyspnea, gasping, apnea
Ocular	Mydriasis, miosis, lacrimation, ptosis, nystagmus, cycloplegia, pupillary light reflex
Gastrointestinal, gastrourinary	Salivation, retching, diarrhea, bloody stool and urine, constipation, rhinorrhea, emesis, involuntary urination and defecation
Cutaneous	Alopecia, piloerection, wet dog shakes, erythema, edema, necrosis, swelling

Source: McNamara, 1976.

value itself has a zero deviation. However, to avoid negative numbers, the probit units are obtained by adding five to these deviations. The corresponding figures in these systems are as follows:

Deviations	Probit	% Response
−3	2	0.1
−2	3	2.3
−1	4	15.9
0	5	50.0
1	6	84.1
2	7	97.7
3	8	99.9

It should be noted that sometimes a more nearly linear relation exists between the probit and the dose expressed arithmetically or with a power function. Detailed methods for estimating the LD_{50} and its standard errors are given in many papers and books on statistics, including those of Bliss (1957), Finney (1971), Litchfield and Wilcox (1949), and Weil (1952); these are therefore not described here.

   Relative Potency   The potency of a toxicant varies significantly. Table 8-2 illustrates the range of LD_{50} values.

   To render the LD_{50} values more meaningful, it is advisable to determine also their standard errors (or the confidence limits) and the slopes of the dose-response curves. If the confidence limits of two LD_{50}s overlap, the substance with a smaller LD_{50} may not be more toxic than the other. The importance of the slope can be readily appreciated when comparing two substances with similar LD_{50}s. The one with a flatter shape will likely cause more deaths than the other at doses smaller than the LD_{50}s (Fig. 8-1, chemicals C and D). The examples in Table 8-3 illustrate the marked differences in slopes.

Uses of LD_{50} Values

These values are useful in a number of ways:

   1   Classification of chemicals according to relative toxicity. A common classification is as follows:

Category	LD_{50}
Supertoxic	5 mg/kg or less
Extremely toxic	5–50 mg/kg
Highly toxic	50–500 mg/kg
Moderately toxic	0.5–5 g/kg
Slightly toxic	5–15 g/kg
Practically nontoxic	>15 g/kg

   2   Evaluation of the hazard from accidental overdosage
   3   Planning subacute and chronic toxicity studies in animals
   4   Providing information about
       (*a*) The mechanism of toxicity
       (*b*) The influence of age, sex, and other host and environmental factors
       (*c*) The variations in response among different animal species and strains
   5   Providing information about the reactivity of a particular animal population
   6   Contributing to the overall information required in planning therapeutic trials of drugs in humans
   7   Quality control of chemicals, to detect toxic impurities and physical chemical changes affecting bioavailability

Table 8-2   Acute LD_{50} Values for a Variety of Chemical Agents

Agent	Species	LD_{50} (mg/kg body weight)
Ethanol	Mouse	10,000
Sodium chloride	Mouse	4,000
Ferrous sulphate	Rat	1,500
Morphine sulphate	Rat	900
Phenobarbital, sodium	Rat	150
DDT	Rat	100
Picrotoxin	Rat	5
Strychnine sulphate	Rat	2
Nicotine	Rat	1
d-Tubocurarine	Rat	0.5
Hemicholinium-3	Rat	0.2
Tetrodotoxin	Rat	0.1
Dioxin (TCDD)	Guinea pig	0.001
Botulinum toxin	Rat	0.00001

Source: Loomis, 1978.

Guidelines for acute oral, dermal, and inhalation toxicity studies have been published by the U.S. Environmental Protection Agency (EPA, 1982).

SHORT-TERM TOXICITY STUDIES

Humans are more often exposed to chemicals at levels much lower than those that are acutely fatal, but they are exposed over longer periods of time. To assess the nature of the toxic effects under these more realistic situations, short-term and long-term toxicity studies are conducted.

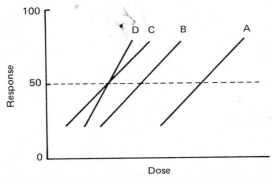

Figure 8-1 Median lethal doses and slopes of the dose-response (death) relationships of four chemicals. Chemical A is less toxic than the others. Chemical C is as toxic as D at the median lethal dose level but is more toxic at lower dose levels. Chemical B is less toxic than D at the median lethal dose level, but it may be more or less so at lower doses.

Table 8-3 Dose-response Relationships[*]

Aflatoxin B$_1$ [†]		Botulinum toxin[‡]			
Dose ppb	Response (tumor)	Dose pg	Response (death)	Dose pg	Response (death)
0	0/18	1	0/10	34	11/30
1	2/22	5	0/10	37	10/30
5	1/22	10	0/30	40	16/30
15	4/21	15	0/30	45	26/30
50	20/25	20	0/30	50	26/30
100	28/28	24	0/30	55	17/30
		27	0/30	60	22/30
		30	4/30	65	20/30

[*]Note relatively shallow dose-response relationship with alfatoxin B$_1$ wherein a 100-fold increase existed between the minimal and maximal effective doses, in contrast to the steep slope of botulinus toxin, wherein there was a mere 50% increase.

[†]Data quoted from Food Safety Council (1980).

[‡]Data supplied by E. J. Schantz (Food Research Institute, University of Wisconsin, Madison, WI 53706). Part of the data also appears in the Report of Food Safety Council (1980).

Experimental Design

Species and Number Generally, two or more species of animals are used. Ideally, the animals chosen should biotransform the chemical in a manner essentially identical to humans. Since this is often unattainable, the rat and the dog are usually selected. This preference is based on their appropriate size, ready availability, and the great preponderance of toxicologic information on chemicals in these animals.

(Equal numbers of male and female animals should be used. Generally, 10–30 rats are used in each dose group as well as in the control group. As a rule, (this procedure will provide data that are statistically analyzable.) Smaller numbers of dogs (4–8 per group) are used because of the greater number of examinations that can be made on each animal and because of their size and the expense involved.

Route of Administration (The chemical should be administered by the route of the intended use or exposure in humans.) For most chemicals, the common route is oral. The preferred procedure is to incorporate the chemical in the diet, although the drinking water is sometimes used as the vehicle. The latter method is advisable when the chemical may react with a component in the diet. The chemical may be administered by gavage or in gelatin capsules, a procedure more often used in dogs. The daily dose of the chemical may also be incorporated in a bolus of canned dog food.

Dermal application, exposure by inhalation, and parenteral routes are used for special purposes, e.g., industrial and agricultural products and drugs.

Dosage and Duration Since the aims of these studies are to determine the nature and site of the toxic effects as well as the "no-effect level," it is advisable to select three doses; a dose that is high enough to elicit definite signs of toxicity but not high enough to kill many of the animals, a low dose that is expected to induce no toxic effect, and an intermediate dose. Sometimes, one or more additional doses are included to ensure that the above objectives are achieved. As noted earlier, a control group should be included. These animals will not receive the chemical under test but must be given any vehicle used.

The doses are generally selected on the basis of the information obtained in the acute toxicity studies, using both the LD_{50} and the slope of the dose-response curve. Any information on related chemicals and on its metabolism, especially the presence or absence of bioaccumulation, is also taken into account.

A range finding study has been proposed. It consists of feeding five rats of each sex at each of three or four dose levels for 7 days. The criteria for toxic effects were mortality, body weight gain, relative liver and kidney weights, and feed consumption. The results indicated that the 7-day tests were considerably better than the LD_{50} values in predicting the dose levels for the 90-day toxicity study (Weil et al., 1969).

In studies in rats, the dose levels may be constant concentrations and expressed in mg/kg diet (ppm) or constant dosage and expressed in mg/kg body weight of the animals. As the animal grows, there are changes in the body weight as well as in the food consumption. For the constant dose regimen, the concentration of the chemical must therefore be adjusted periodically to maintain a relatively constant dose in mg/kg body weight. This is usually done at weekly intervals during the period of rapid growth and biweekly thereafter.

The duration of such studies in rats is generally 90 days. In the dog, the duration is often extended to 6 months or even 1 or 2 years.

Observations and Examinations

Body Weight and Food Consumption These should be determined weekly. Decreased body weight gain is a simple yet sensitive index of toxic effects. Food consumption is also a useful indicator. In addition, a marked decrease in food consumption can induce effects that mimic or aggravate the toxic manifestations of the chemical. In such cases, paired feeding or parenteral feeding may have to be instituted.

General Observations (These should include appearance, behavior, and any abnormality.) Dead and moribund animals should be removed from the cages for gross and possibly microscopic examination. Frequent observation is necessary to minimize cannibalism.

Laboratory Tests *Hematologic* examinations usually include hematocrit, hemoglobin, erythrocyte count, total leukocyte count, and differential leukocyte count. All dogs should be sampled before the initiation of treatment and at one week, one month, and at the end. Tests at other intervals may be warranted. Because of the small blood volume of rats, only half of them are sampled at various intervals, while the others only at the end. Speical tests such as reticulocyte count, platelet count, methemoglobin, and glucose-6-phosphate dehydrogenase (G-6-PD) may be indicated.

Clinical laboratory tests usually include fasting blood glucose, serum glutamic oxalacetic acid transaminase (SGOT), serum glutamic pyruvic acid transaminase (SGPT), alkaline phosphatase, total protein, albumin, globulin, blood urea nitrogen (BUN), and such elements as sodium, potassium, calcium, and phosphorus.

Urinalysis usually includes color, specific gravity, pH, protein, glucose, ketones, formed elements (red blood cells, etc.), and crystalline and amorphous materials. Additional details of these laboratory tests and a variety of special tests for assessing damages to target organs are provided in the proceedings of the Workshop on Subchronic Toxicity (1980).

Postmortem Examination Whenever possible, all animals that are found dead or dying should be subjected to a gross pathologic examination. If the state of the tissue permits, histologic examinations should also be done. In addition, the weights of a number of organs, either in absolute values or in terms of the body weights, should be determined as they serve as useful indicators of toxicity.

The organs that are usually weighed are liver, kidneys, adrenals, heart, brain, thyroid, and testes or ovaries. Those that are histologically examined are the following: all gross lesions, brain (3 levels), spinal cord, eye and optic nerve, a major salivary gland, thymus, thyroid, heart, aorta, lung with a bronchus, stomach, small intestine (3 levels), large intestine (2 levels), adrenal gland, pancreas, liver, gallbladder (if present), spleen, kidney, urinary bladder, skeletal muscle, bone and its marrow.

A list indicating the correlation between general observations, clinical laboratory tests, and postmortem examinations is reproduced as Table 8-4.

Guidelines for short-term oral, dermal, and inhalation studies have been published by the U.S. Environmental Protection Agency (EPA, 1982).

Evaluation

A comprehensive short-term toxicity study, using the various parameters of observations and examinations described above, usually will yield information on the toxicity of the chemical under test, with respect to the target organs, the effects on these organs, and the dose-effect and dose-response relationships.

Table 8-4 General Observations, Clinical Laboratory Tests, and Pathology Examinations that may be used in Subchronic Toxicity Studies

Organ or organ system	General observations	Clinical laboratory tests on blood	Pathology examination [*]
Liver	Discoloration of mucus membranes, edema, ascites	Glutamic oxaloacetic transaminase (GOT), glutamic pyruvate transaminase, alkaline phosphatase (AP), cholesterol, total protein, albumin, globulin	Liver[†]
Gastrointestinal (GI) system	Diarrhea, vomit, stool, appetite	Total protein, albumin, globulin, sodium (Na), potassium (K)	Stomach, GI tract, gall-bladder (if present), salivary gland, pancreas
Urinary system	Urine volume, consistency, color	Blood urea nitrogen, total protein, albumin, globulin	Kidney and urinary bladder[†]
Hematopoietic/ hemostatic system	Discoloration of mucous membranes, lethargy, weakness	Packed red cell volume, hemoglobin, erythrocyte count, total and differential leukocyte count, thrombocyte count, blood smear, prothrombin time, activated partial thromboplastin time	Spleen, thymus, mesenteric lymph nodes, bone marrow smear and section
Nervous system	Posture, movements, responses, behavior		Brain, spinal cord, and sciatic nerve
Eye	Appearance, discharge, ophthalmologic examination		Eye and optic nerves
Respiratory system	Rate, coughing, nasal discharge	Total protein, albumin, globulin	One lung with a major bronchus
Endocrine system	Skin, hair coat, body weight, urine and stool characteristics	Glucose, Na, K, AP (dog), cholesterol	Thyroid, adrenal, pancreas
Reproductive system	Appearance and palpation of external reproductive organs		Testes and epididymis or ovaries. Uterus or prostate and seminal vesicles[†]
Skeletal system	Growth, deformation, lameness	Calcium, phosphorus, AP	Bone and breakage strength
Cardiovascular system	Rate and characteristic of pulse, rhythm, edema, ascites	GOT	Heart,[†] aorta, small arteries in other tissues
Skin	Color, appearance, odor, hair coat	Total protein, albumin, globulin	Only in dermal studies
Muscle	Size, weakness, wasting, decreased activity	GOT, creatine phosphokinase	Only if indicated by observations, clinical chemistry or gross lesions

Source: Workshop on Subchronic Toxicity Testing, 1980.
[*]All animals should undergo thorough gross examination; organs or tissues listed should be examined microscopically.
[†]These organs should also be weighed.

Such information often provides indication on the additional specific types of studies that should be conducted. The quantitative data from the short-term and other studies have been suggested for use in the determination of the "no-effect level" (NEL). However, this suggestion has not been widely accepted (e.g., Gehring and Rao, 1979).

For certain types of chemicals, the NEL from short-term studies, along with data on their acute toxicity and metabolism as well as information from genetic, reproductive, and any other studies, is used in determining their "acceptable intakes" for humans. For further discussion on the procedure used for this purpose, see "Long-Term Toxicity Studies."

LONG-TERM TOXICITY STUDIES

Experimental Design

Animals: Species and Number Generally one or more species of animals are used. Unless otherwise indicated the rat is used; dogs and nonhuman primates are next in preference. Because of their small size, mice are not suitable for long-term general toxicity studies, although they are often used in carcinogenesis studies.

An equal number of male and female animals should be used. Generally 40–100 rats are placed in each dose group and in the control group. Much smaller numbers of dogs and nonhuman primates are used.

Route of Administration and Dosage and Duration Route of administration is the same as in short-term studies. The criteria for the selection of doses are the same as in short-term studies. But because of the considerable time and expense involved in conducting such studies, greater care should be taken in selecting the doses.

The duration of such studies in rats is usually 2 years. Some investigators advocate even longer duration, which is increasingly feasible. However, because of complication with signs of senility, it is generally recommended that the duration should not exceed 30 months. Dogs and monkeys are kept for 6 years or more.

Observations and Examinations

These should include body weight, food consumption, general observations, laboratory tests, and postmortem examinations, as described under short-term studies.

Guidelines on the testing procedures and on the interpretation of the results are included in certain WHO publications (e.g., WHO, 1958; 1974; 1978). Guidelines have been published by the U.S. Environmental Protection Agency (EPA, 1982).

Evaluation

The purposes of the long-term toxicity study are to define the nature of the toxicity of the chemical and to determine the NEL. The procedures for these are described in Chapter 7.

If the nature of the toxicity is not serious, and an NEL has been demonstrated, an acceptable intake can be extrapolated from the animal data. This is generally done by the application of a safety factor. This factor allows partly for any differences in sensitivity between the animal species and humans, partly for the wide variations in sensitivity among the human population, and partly for the fact that the number of animals tested is small compared with the size of the human population that may be exposed. Additional details are provided in Chapter 7.

A safety factor of 100 has long been recommended (WHO, 1958) and has been widely accepted; however, this figure is not invariably applied. For example, when toxicologic data derived from critical observations in humans are available, a lower safety factor may be justified. On the other hand, a larger safety factor may be used where the amount and/or the quality of the toxicologic information is somewhat limited. This is also true with the chemicals that produce more serious toxic effects at the higher dose levels.

As our understanding of toxicology expands, more and more types of observations and examinations are being included in the protocol of long-term studies. In spite of this trend, a variety of specific studies have been designed to elucidate the nature of the toxicity and the mechanism of action of chemicals. These special studies should be undertaken wherever indicated. Such indications may arise from the chemical nature of the substance or from the experimental findings in the short-term and long-term studies. The results of such specific studies can have a bearing on the size of the safety factor used in arriving at an acceptable daily intake (ADI), and they can even have an impact on the decision as to whether or not an ADI should be allocated.

REFERENCES

Balazs, T. (1976) Assessment of the value of systemic toxicity studies. In: *New Concepts in Safety Evaluation*. Eds. M. A. Mehlman, R. E. Shapiro, and H. Blumenthal. Washington, D.C.: Hemisphere.

Bliss, C. L. (1957) Some principles of bioassay. *Am. Sci.* 45:449–466.

EPA (1982) *Health Effects Test Guidelines. Hazard Evaluation. EPA 560/6-82-001.* Springfield, Va.: National Technical Information Service (NTIS No. PB82-232984).

Ferguson, H. C. (1962) Dilution of dose and acute oral toxicity. *Toxicol. Appl. Pharmacol.* 4:759.

Finney, D. J. (1971) *Probit Analysis.* Cambridge: Cambridge Univ. Press.

Food Safety Council (1980) *Proposed System for Food Safety Assessment.* Washington, D.C.: Food Safety Council.

Gehring, P. J., and Rao, K. S. (1979) Toxicologic data extrapolation. In: *Patty's Industrial Hygiene and Toxicology*. Eds. L. V. Cralley and L. J. Cralley. New York: John Wiley.

Griffith, J. F. (1964) Interlaboratory variations in the determination of the acute oral LD_{50}. *Toxicol. Appl. Pharmacol.* 6:726–730.

Litchfield, J. T., and Wilcoxom, F. (1949) A simplified method of evaluating dose-effect experiments. *J. Pharmacol. Exp. Ther.* 96:90–113.

Loomis, T. (1978) *Essentials of Toxicology*, 3d ed. Philadelphia: Lea & Febiger.

Lu, F. C., Jessup, D. C., and Lavallee, A. (1965) Toxicity of pesticides in young versus adult rats. *Food Cosmet. Toxicol.* 3:591–596.

McNamara, B. P. (1976) Concepts in health evaluation of commercial and industrial chemicals. In: *New Concepts in Safety Evaluation*. Eds. M. A. Mehlman, R. E. Shapiro, and H. Blumenthal. Washington, D.C.: Hemisphere.

Sperling, F. (1976) Non-lethal parameters as indices of acute toxicity: Inadequacy of the acute LD_{50}. In: *New Concepts in Safety Evaluation*. Eds. M. A. Mehlman, R. E. Shapiro, and H. Blumenthal. Washington, D.C.: Hemisphere.

Weil, C. S. (1952) Tables for convenient calculation of median effective dose (LD_{50} or ED_{50}) and instructions for their use. *Biometrics* 8:249–263.

Weil, C. S., Carpenter, C. F., and Smyth, H. F., Jr. (1953) Specifications for calculating the median effective dose. *Am. Ind. Hyg. Assoc. J.* 14:200–206.

Weil, C. S., Woodside, M. D., Bernard, J. R., and Carpenter, C. P. (1969) Relationship between single-peroral, one-week and 90-day rat feeding studies. *Toxicol. Appl. Pharmacol.* 14:426–431.

WHO (1958) *Second Report of the Expert Committee on Food Additives*. WHO Tech. Rep. Ser. No. 144. Geneva: World Health Organization.

WHO (1974) *Seventeenth Report of the Expert Committee on Food Additives*. WHO Tech. Rep. Ser. No. 539. Geneva: World Health Organization.

WHO (1978) *Principles and Methods for Evaluating the Toxicity of Chemicals, Part I*, Environmental Health Criteria 6. Geneva: World Health Organization.

Workshop on Subchronic Toxicity Testing (1980) *Proceedings of the Workshop EPA-560/11-80-028*. Eds. N. Page, D. Sawbney, and M. G. Ryon. Springfield, Va.: National Technical Information Service.

Chapter 9

Carcinogenesis

INTRODUCTION

In many countries, cancer is one of the leading causes of death. It is induced by a variety of agents, the most important being certain life styles, e.g., smoking cigarettes, drinking alcoholic beverages, chewing betal. However, chemicals in the community and workplace and some therapeutic agents also play a role. Attempts at reducing cancer incidence are therefore aimed at reducing these hazardous life styles as well as at identifying these chemical carcinogens, in the hope that human exposure to them can be eliminated or minimized. Table 9-1 is a list of chemicals that are considered as definite or probable human carcinogens (IARC, 1979).

Another type of research in carcinogenesis is aimed at improving existing methods and devising new methods for prompt and reliable identification of carcinogenic chemicals. Presently available methods are either too costly and time-consuming or are not adequately reliable. This problem stems mainly from the fact that cancer only occurs in response to a chemical long after its first entry into an organism. Often the chemical is no longer detectable in the body by the time the tumor develops.

113

Table 9-1   Carcinogenic Chemicals

The Working Group concluded that the following chemicals, groups of chemicals, and industrial processes are *carcinogenic for humans* (Group 1):

4-Aminobiphenyl	Cyclophosphamide[†]
Arsenic and certain arsenic compounds	Furniture and cabinet-making industry
Asbestos	(certain industries)[†]
Manufacture of auramine[*]	Underground hematite mining[*]
Benzene	Manufacture of isopropyl alcohol by the
Benzidine	strong acid process[*]
N,N-bis(2-chloroethyl)-2-naphthylamine	Melphalan
(chlornaphazine)	Mustard gas
Bis(chloromethyl)ether and technical	2-Naphthylamine
grade chloromethyl methyl ether	Nickel refining[*]
Boot and shoe manufacturing and repair	Soots, tars, and mineral oils[*]
(certain industries)[†]	Vinyl chloride
Chromium and certain chromium	
compounds[*]	
Conjugated estrogens[†]	

The following 18 chemicals and groups of chemicals are *probably carcinogenic for humans* (Group 2):

Group A (5 chemicals)

Aflatoxins	Nickel and certain nickel compounds[*]
Cadmium and certain cadmium compounds[*]	Tris(1-aziridinyl)phosphine sulphide
Chlorambucil	(thiotepa)

Group B (12 chemicals)

Acrylonitrile	Dimethylsulphate
Amitrole (aminotriazole)	Ethylene oxide
Auramine	Iron dextran
Beryllium and certain beryllium compounds[*]	Oxymetholone
Carbon tetrachloride	Phenacetin
Dimethylcarbamoyl chloride	Polychlorinated biphenyls

Source: IARC Monographs for Carcinogenic Chemicals, 1979, Vol. 1–20, Supplement 1.

[†]These chemicals have been added from Vol. 21–25.

[*]The specific compound(s) that may be responsible for a carcinogenic effect in humans cannot be specified precisely.

In addition, the evaluation of the health hazards of such chemicals is a complex matter. First, the effects of certain carcinogens are persistent. Second, there are several categories of carcinogens with different mechanisms of action. Thus they pose different health hazards and this fact must be taken into account in their evaluation.

Definition

The therm *chemical carcinogenesis* is generally defined to indicate the induction or enhancement of neoplasia by chemicals. Although in the strict etymologic sense this term means the induction of carcinomas, it is widely used to indicate tumorigenesis. In other words, it includes not only epithelial malignancies (carcinomas) but also mesenchymal malignant tumors (sarcomas) and benign tumors. The extension to benign tumor is justified because no real carcinogen that produces only benign tumors has been discovered.

It is generally agreed (e.g., WHO, 1969) that the response of an organism to a carcinogen may be in one or more of these forms:

1. An increase in the frequency of one or several types of tumors that also occur in the controls
2. The development of tumors not seen in the controls
3. The occurrence of tumors earlier than in the controls
4. An increase in the number of tumors in individual animals, compared to the controls

Mode of Action

Chemical carcinogenesis, as shown in Fig. 9-1, is a multistage process. Carcinogenic chemicals act either by covalently binding with genetic macromolecules or by promoting the process. The former type of chemicals are known as genotoxic carcinogens because they, or their reactive metabolites, react with the genetic materials.

After the interaction between a genotoxic carcinogen and the DNA, the affected cell either dies or reverts to a normal cell through error-free DNA repair. If neither of these events occurs, the carcinogenic initiation becomes irreversible after the cell undergoes replication. Such an initiated cell may remain dormant for a long period of time before it becomes a tumor through cellular proliferation.

Initiated cells remain dormant probably because of the suppressant influence of the surrounding normal cells. This influence is apparently reduced under a number of conditions. These include cell removal (e.g., partial hepatectomy), cell killing (resulting from cytotoxic chemicals, viruses, radiation), growth factors (e.g., hormones), and exogenous factors (see Trosko and Chang, 1983).

Epigenetic carcinogens increase the tumor yield by promoting the replication of cells initiated by genotoxic carcinogens, or by augmenting the available amount of genotoxic carcinogens and/or their metabolites at the site of action. In long-term carcinogenesis studies, the animals given epigenetic carcinogens develop more tumors than the controls, or the tumors appear earlier, presumably because of promotion of neoplastic cells arising from inherited genetic defects or from exposure to unknown environmental genotoxic carcinogens. The various mechanisms of action of epigenetic carcinogens are outlined in the following section.

CLASSIFICATION

Chemical carcinogens can be classified according to the strength of their potency. Potent carcinogens, e.g., aflatoxins and certain nitrosamines, produce a high

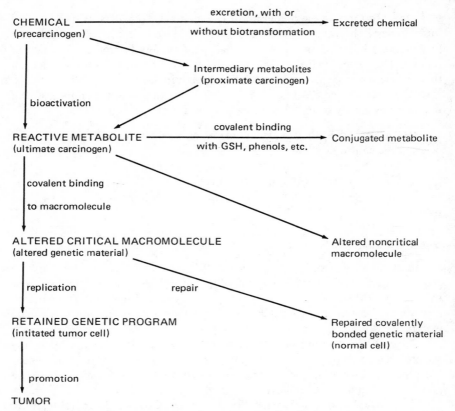

Figure 9-1 Schematic diagram depicting the fate of a genetic carcinogen and its relation with tumorigenesis (adapted from Gehring et al., 1979). Events in left-hand column lead to tumor formation, whereas those in right-hand column are harmless.

incidence of cancers in small-scale animal experiments, even at low dose levels. On the other hand, weak carcinogens require a large population of experimental animals given large doses to reveal their carcinogenic effects.

The quality and quantity of the available *information* have also been used in classifying carcinogens. One such scheme places carcinogens in the following categories: (1) recognized or proved carcinogens refer to those with activity established in epidemiologic studies or with other types of strong evidence; (2) suspect carcinogens are those with suggestive but not conclusive evidence; (3) potential carcinogens include substances with chemical structures similar to proved carcinogens but not yet tested; and (4) inadequate data for classification (Kraybill, 1977).

They may also be classified according to their *mode of action* into genotoxic and epigenetic (nongenotoxic) carcinogens (Weisburger and Williams, 1980; ICPEPC, 1982).

Genotoxic Carcinogens

Genotoxic carcinogens initiate tumors by producing DNA damage through covalent binding (Fig. 9-1). There are two types.

The *direct-acting carcinogens* (also known as ultimate carcinogens) are electrophilic and can bind to DNA and other macromolecules. Examples are alkyl and aryl epoxides, lactones, sulfate esters, nitrosamides, and nitrosoureas.

The *precarcinogens* (also known as procarcinogens) require conversion through bioactivation to become ultimate carcinogens, either directly or via an intermediary stage, the proximate carcinogens. Most of the presently known chemical carcinogens fall into this class. These include the polynuclear aromatic hydrocarbons (PAH), aromatic amines, nitrosamines, aflatoxin B, pyrrolizidine alkaloids, safrole, cycasin, and thioamides. Different types of bioactivations are involved in their conversion to the direct-acting agents, as discussed in Chapter 3.

There are pure initiators, such as trans-4-acetyl-aminostilbene, which can convert normal cells but cannot, in the absence of promoters, produce tumors. Complete genotoxic carcinogens, such as 2-AAF, act as initiator and promoter (Neumann, 1983).

Epigenetic Carcinogens

These substances do not damage DNA but enhance the growth of tumors induced by genotoxic carcinogens. There are different modes of action.

Cocarcinogens enhance the effects of genotoxic carcinogens when given simultaneously. They may act by effecting an increase in the concentration of the initiator, the genotoxic carcinogen itself, or that of the reactive metabolite. This can be achieved either by an increase of the absorption of the carcinogen, via the gastrointestinal tract or the skin, or by an increase of the bioactivation. The same result can also be achieved through a decrease of the elimination of the initiator either by inhibiting the detoxification enzymes or by depleting the endogenous substrates involved in Phase II reactions, such as glutathione. Other cocarcinogens such as ferric oxide and asbestos probably facilitate cellular uptake of genotoxic carcinogens.

Apart from increasing the concentration of the reactive species at the site of action, cocarcinogens may inhibit the rate or fidelity of DNA repair, or they may enhance conversion of DNA lesions to permanent alterations (see Williams, 1984).

Promoters increase the effects of initiators when given subsequently. The classic example of this phenomenon was provided by studies demonstrating that an initial application on mouse skin of a carcinogenic PAH did not induce skin cancer until after applying, at the same site, phorbol esters from croton oil (Berenblum and Shubik, 1947; 1949). The application of the promoters could be delayed for months or even a year without losing the effect. These studies clearly demonstrate the *two-stage* process of carcinogenesis as well as the persistence of the effect of the initiator. Incidentally, croton oil is also cocarcinogenic since it is effective when applied at the same time as the initiator.

The possible mechanisms of action of promoters include: (1) stimulation of cell proliferation through cytoxicity or hormonal effects; (2) inhibition of intercellular communication, thereby releasing the initiated cells from the restraint exercised by the surrounding normal cells; and (3) immunosuppression. Thus, among the promoters are two special groups of chemicals, namely hormones and immunosuppressive drugs.

Hormones such as estradiol and diethylstilbestrol have been shown to cause an increase in tumors in animals (e.g., breast cancer in mice) and in humans (e.g., endometrial cancer in menopausal females maintained on estrogen). These substances are not genotoxic but act as promoters. The actual initiators are not known. Androgens have little, if any, carcinogenic effect.

Immunosuppressive drugs are increasingly being used in conjunction with organ transplantation. They have been shown to cause leukemias and sarcomas in some of these patients and in mice and rats. The genotoxic agents are likely to be viruses, and the immunosuppressive drugs promote the development of the tumors through epigenetic mechanisms.

Solid-state carcinogens are exemplified by asbestos and implanted materials such as plastics, metal, and glass. These substances show no genotoxicity, and they produce tumors of mesenchymal origin. While the precise mode of action is not known, the tumors they induce is preceded by an exuberant foreign body reaction with a high frequency of chromosomal changes in the preneoplastic cells (Rachko and Brand, 1983).

Table 9-2 provides a comparison of initiating agents and promoting agents.

Others

A number of *metals and metalloids* (e.g., arsenic, chromium, and nickel) and their compounds are carcinogenic in animals; some of them are considered to be carcinogens in humans also (IARC, 1979). Arsenic was thought to be an exception in that it is carcinogenic in humans but not in animals. Recent data, however, show that intratracheal instillation of AsO_3 in Syrian hamsters, resulted in an increase in pulmonary adenomas, and after intrauterine exposure, it apparently caused lung tumors in mice. Nevertheless, arsenic appears to be different from chromium, nickel, and others, in that it is not mutagenic per se in bacterial systems but merely blocks the excision repair induced by other mutagenic agents. It has therefore been considered a co-mutagen. On the other hand, a number of metals are mutagenic in bacterial systems. The results in such

Table 9-2 Comparison of Biologic Properties of Initiating Agents and Promoting Agents

Initiating agents	Promoting agents
1. Carcinogenic by themselves "solitary carcinogens"	1. Not carcinogenic alone
2. Must be given before promoting agent	2. Must be given after initiating agent
3. Single exposure is sufficient	3. Require prolonged exposure
4. Action is "irreversible" and additive	4. Action is reversible (at early stage) and not additive
5. No apparent threshold	5. Probable threshold
6. Yield electrophiles—bind covalently to cell macromolecules	6. No evidence of covalent binding
7. Mutagenic	7. Not mutagenic

Source: Weinstein, 1980; p. 91.

systems and those obtained from other in vitro tests have been summarized by Sunderman (1984) and are reproduced in Table 9-3.

With respect to the mechanisms of metal carcinogenesis, Sunderman (1984) has listed the following as the most promising avenues for research: The metal cations (1) covalently bind to DNA, (2) form cross-links between DNA and proteins or between adjacent DNA strands, (3) impair the fidelity of DNA replication by altering the conformation of DNA polymerases, (4) cause helical transition from B-DNA to Z-DNA, affecting chromatin structure, and (5) bind to histones, nonhistone nuclear proteins, or nucleolar RNA, influencing chromatin structure and gene expression. These substances may be classified as genotoxic carcinogens since they alter the gene expression in one way or another.

The term *secondary carcinogens* has been used to refer to substances that are not directly carcinogenic but can induce cancer following a distinctly non-carcinogenic effect. For example, polyoxyethylene monostearate (Myrj 45), at very high doses, elicited bladder stones that in turn caused bladder tumors. No tumors were observed in any of the animals that had no bladder stones. On the other hand, this term has also been used in connection with those genotoxic carcinogens that require bioactivation.

LONG-TERM CARCINOGENICITY STUDIES

These studies are designed to provide definitive information on the carcinogenic effects of chemicals on the test animals. Because of the great expense and time required, they are undertaken usually after a review of other data, such as the chemical structure and results from short-term mutagenesis tests and long-term chronic toxicity studies, which are described, respectively, in a following section and in Chapter 8.

Guidelines on the long-term carcinogenicity studies are outlined in this

Table 9-3 In Vitro Experiments Related to Carcinogenesis

Experimental system	Metals whose compounds have yielded positive results																
	Ag	As	Be	Cd	Co	Cr	Cu	Fe	Hg	Mn	Ni	Pb	Pt	Sb	Sn	Tl	Zn
Mutagenesis and recassays in bacteria	X	?	X	X	X	X		X	X	X	X		X	X		X	X
Mutagenesis in mammalian cells	X	X	X	X	X	X	X	X	X	X	X	X	X				X
Chromosomal damage and sister chromatid exchanges		X	X		X	X			X	X	X	X	X				X
Morphologic transformation	X	X	X	X	X	X	X	X	X	X	X	X	X	X		X	X
DNA strandbreaks, DNA-protein cross-links	X			X	X	X	X				X		X		X		
DNA polymerase infidelity	X		X	X	X	X	X			X	X	X					
RNA strand initiation			X	X	X					X	X	X					
Conversion of B-DNA to Z-DNA					X					X	X						

Source: Sunderman, 1984.

section. More detailed descriptions and references to some comments are provided in a paper (Page, 1977) and in three publications (WHO, 1978; IARC, 1980a; and OECD, 1981).

Animals: Species, Strain, Sex, and Number

Rats and mice are generally preferred because of their small size, short life-span, ready availability, and an abundance of information on their response to other carcinogens. Hamsters are also used, especially in studies on cancers of the bladder, breast, gastrointestinal tract, and respiratory tract (e.g., for tobacco smoke). Dogs and nonhuman primates are occasionally used, the former for their positive response to 4-aminobiphenyl and 2-naphthylamine and the latter for their higher phylogenetic order. But their use is limited because of their large size and relatively long life-span, thereby requiring a 7- to 10-year exposure to the chemical on test.

The characteristics of a preferred strain are (1) known sensitivity to substances of similar chemical structure, (2) low incidence of spontaneous tumors, and (3) similarity of its rate and pattern of biotransformation and those of humans, if known.

Highly inbred strains should not be used to avoid possible insensitivity. Hybrid mice of two known inbred strains are preferable because they lack the possible insensitivity of inbred strains and they are generally more robust.

Both sexes should be included in these studies; differences in response to the carcinogenic activity of chemicals are well documented.

To provide a sufficient number of animals surviving till the appearance of tumors for statistical analysis, it is a common practice to start the tests with 50 animals of each sex per dose group, including the controls.

Inception and Duration

The studies are generally started shortly after weaning the animals to allow maximum duration of exposure. The use of neonates is not generally recommended because of their differences from weanling and adult animals in metabolic capability, anatomic and physiologic characteristics, viral susceptibility, hormonal status, and immunologic competence. Multigeneration studies and the use of pregnant animals for exposure of the embryo or the fetus in utero have been used, but their advantages and drawbacks need further investigation.

The duration of the studies is generally 24 months in rats and 18 months in mice. If the animals are in good condition, the duration may be extended to 30 and 24 months, respectively.

Route of Administration

The chemical under test should be given to the animals by the route of human exposure. This principle readily applies to food additives and contaminants as well as most drugs. However, for industrial and environmental chemicals, the main route of entry is inhalation. Because of lack of adequate facilities, such chemicals have usually been tested by the oral route. When this is done, however, the kinetics of the chemical by the oral and the inhalation routes must be compared to ensure appropriate extrapolation of the data from one route to the other. Alternatively, the test chemical may be instilled intratracheally.

When the test substance is to be given orally, it can be mixed with the diet, either in constant concentration (in milligrams of the chemical per kilogram diet, ppm) or in constant dosage (in milligrams of the chemical per kilogram of body weight). In the latter case, it is necessary to adjust the concentration of the chemical in the diet according to the food consumption and the body weight at appropriate intervals. The chemical may also be incorporated in the drinking water instead of the diet, or it may be given by gavage.

Commercial animal feed may contain small amounts of carcinogens (e.g., aflatoxins) or enzyme inducers (e.g., DDT), which can modify the effects of the test chemical.

Dermal application is used for industrial chemicals and drugs intended for topical use. This route is mainly intended for detecting local carcinogenicity. However, in some cases, appreciable amounts may be absorbed to induce systemic effects. The choice of vehicle is important: it ought to have little or no toxicity per se and should not react with the chemical under test. Dimethyl sulfoxide is often used.

Parenteral administration by intravenous, intraperitoneal, or subcutaneous injection is used only rarely and only when there is special reason for selecting these routes. These routes are impractical and their results may be complicated by local reactions.

Doses

Usually two or three dose levels are included in such studies. In addition, control groups are also included for comparison. The doses are selected on the basis of the short-term studies and metabolism data, with the aim that the high dose would produce some minor signs of toxicity but not significantly reduce the lifespan of the animals. The two lower doses are generally some fractions of the high dose (e.g., $\frac{1}{2}$ and $\frac{1}{4}$) and are expected to permit the animals to survive in good health or until tumor develops.

The National Cancer Institute (1976) proposed the use of the "maximally tolerated dose" (MTD) as the high dose. It is estimated from 90-day studies and defined as one that would (1) cause no more than 10% weight decrement compared to the controls and (2) not induce death nor produce any clinical signs of toxicity or pathologic lesions that would shorten the life-span of the animal.

In general, these criteria appear satisfactory for the selection of the dose levels. However, with certain chemicals, as discussed in a subsequent section, there may be extensive organ damage or overloading of the normal biotransformation mechanism at such doses. In these cases, critical evaluation of the results or even repetition of the experiments at lower doses is warranted.

On the other hand, with apparently innocuous substances, the high dose should represent no more than 5% of the diet; if the test substance is a nutrient, a larger percentage may be used.

Controls and Combined Treatment

An untreated group consisting of the same number, or a larger number, of animals as each dose group is included. In addition to these negative controls, another group of animals should be incorporated that should be given a known carcinogen at a dose level that had shown to be carcinogenic. The positive controls provide more confidence in the results on the test chemical by serving as a check on the sensitivity of the particular lot of animals used as well as the adequacy of the facilities and procedures in the specific laboratory. It will also provide some indication of the relative potency of the test chemical. If a vehicle, such as acetone or dimethyl sulfoxide, is to be used, its possible effect should also be tested in a group of animals.

The importance of historical control has been emphasized by the Task Force (1982).

A chemical may be given to the test animals along with a known carcinogen. This is done when the test chemical has a low carcinogenic effect and humans may be exposed to both under realistic situations. This is also done when the test chemical is expected to modify the effects of other environmental carcinogens.

Observations and Examinations

Body Weight and Food Consumption   Body weight and food consumption should be recorded. These figures allow the calculation of the intake of the chemical on a milligram per kilogram body weight basis. Furthermore, the body weight is a sensitive index of the health status of the animal and should be determined at weekly intervals during the first 3 months, when the animals are growing, and biweekly afterward.

General Observations   The animals should be examined daily for mortality and morbidity. Dead and moribund animals should be removed from the cage for gross and microscopic examinations whenever the condition of the tissues permit.

Sick animals should be placed in single cages to prevent cannibalism and for quarantine. If indicated, they may be treated with drugs, but any therapy must be recorded. Prolonged drug treatment should be avoided to preclude possible interference with the effect of the chemical under test.

The onset, location, size, and growth of any unusual tissue masses should be carefully examined and recorded. Signs of toxicity and pharmacologic effects should also be noted.

Laboratory Tests Unlike the short-term and long-term toxicity studies in which all toxic effects are to be investigated, the main purpose of the carcinogenicity studies is to determine the carcinogenic activity of the chemical. Therefore, in the interest of the health of the animals, few tests are performed except the standard hematologic examinations. These are done at the termination of the study. If they are to be done at mid-term, additional animals should be started.

Postmortem Examinations All animals found dead or dying should be subjected to gross autopsy. The survivals at the end of the study should be sacrificed and examined. In addition, a number of organs should be weighed, including the liver, kidneys, heart, testes, and brain.

Samples of all tissues should be preserved for histologic examination. Microscopic examinations should be done on all tumor growths and all tissues showing gross abnormalities. Usually the following tissues are also examined: mandibular lymph node, salivary gland, mammary gland, sternebrae, femor or vertebrae (including marrow), thymus, thyroid, parathyroid, trachea, lungs and main bronchi, heart, esophagus, stomach, small intestine, colon, liver, gallbladder, pancreas, spleen, adrenals, kidneys, urinary bladder, prostate, testes, uterus, ovaries, brain (3 sections), pituitary, eyes (if grossly abnormal), spinal cord (if neurologic signs).

Reporting of Tumors Some of the terms used to describe tumors, e.g., hepatoma, have broad definitions. A detailed description of the pathologic picture of the lesions is thus invaluable.

As carcinogenesis can manifest in a variety of forms (see "Definition"), it is necessary to record the following:

1 The number of various types of tumors (both benign and malignant), and any unusual tumors
2 The number of tumor-bearing animals
3 The number of tumors in each animal
4 The onset of tumors whenever determinable

RAPID SCREENING TESTS

Short-Term Tests for Mutagenesis/Carcinogenesis

In recent years, a number of relatively simple and much shorter tests have been devised and employed to detect the mutagenic activity of chemicals. These tests utilize a variety of systems, including bacteria, cells from plants (e.g., Tradescantia), insects, and isolated mammalian cells, as well as a battery of parameters such as various gene mutation, chromosomal effects, and DNA repair. These mutagenesis tests and short-term carcinogenesis tests using cell transformation as endpoint will be described and discussed in the next chapter.

Although not all mutagens are carcinogenic nor vice versa, the relationship between these two activities is nevertheless so close that mutagenesis tests are performed frequently as a rapid screening of chemicals for their potential carcinogenicity. To improve the reliability of the results, a battery of these tests is usually conducted (IARC, 1980b). Weisburger and Williams (1981) recommended the following short-term in vitro tests: (1) bacterial mutagenesis, (2) mammalian mutagenesis, (3) DNA repair, (4) chromosome damage, and (5) cell transformation.

Limited Carcinogenicity Tests

Limited carcinogenicity tests have been recommended by Weisburger and Williams (1980) and Green et al. (1981), because of certain advantages. These tests are superior to the mutagenesis tests in that the endpoint is tumor formation. Furthermore, the duration of these tests is much shorter than that of the long-term carcinogenicity studies.

Skin Tumor in Mice Mouse skin responds to topical application of chemicals, such as polycyclic aromatic hydrocarbons, and crude products, such as tars from coal and petroleum, by the formation of papillomas and carcinomas. This procedure, introduced by Berenblum and Shubik (1947), has been widely used. Mouse skin responds positively apparently because it has the enzymes that convert the substances into active metabolites.

Some chemicals act as initiator and as promoter; they may therefore be referred to as complete carcinogens. Others act mainly or exclusively as initiators. This carcinogenicity is revealed only after the application of a promoter (Slaga et al., 1982). Results obtained in the mouse skin test reported in the literature on the effects of chemicals as initiators and as promoters have been compiled by Pereira (1982).

Pulmonary Tumor in Mice Strain A mice spontaneously have an essentially 100 percent lung tumor incidence by 24 months of age. Positive results from carcinogens can be obtained in about 24 weeks when few controls have tumors. With some chemicals, the test can be completed in 12 weeks (Shimkin and Stoner, 1975).

Altered Foci in Rodent Liver It has been demonstrated that distinct liver foci appear before the development of hepatocarcinoma. These foci are resistant to iron accumulation, a phenomenon that can be identified histochemically. There are also abnormalities in certain enzymes, which can be demonstrated histochemically. The latter alteration occurs in rats but not in mice. These foci can be detected within 3 weeks of exposure and occur in large numbers in 12–16 weeks (Williams and Watanabe, 1978; Goldfarb and Pugh, 1982).

Breast Cancer in Female Rats Polycyclic hydrocarbons can induce breast cancers in young female Sprague-Dawley and Wister rats. The tumors can develop in less than 6 months (Huggins et al., 1959).

In addition to the above tests, Green et al. (1981) also included such procedures as neonatal exposure, implantation, injection, and intratracheal intubation.

Biochemical Tests

Endoplasmic Reticulum Derangement Svoboda and Reddy (1975) observed that treatment with chemical carcinogens caused structural disorganization of the endoplasmic reticulum within the cells of target tissues. Among the structural changes, degranulation or the detachment of ribosomes from the extravesicular surfaces of the rough endoplasmic reticulum (RER) appeared to be a common effect of chemical carcinogens. In addition, Williams and Parry (1975) have shown that the in vivo degranulatory action of chemical carcinogens could be reproduced in the in vitro situation. Using the in vitro procedure, two groups of investigators have found a good correlation of the RER degranulation in the rat and mouse with the in vivo carcinogenicity in these animals for a number of carcinogenic and noncarcinogenic chemicals tested (see Wright et al., 1977).

Biochemical Marker Biochemical markers for initiation, promotion, and tumor are biochemical tools for the detection of the occurrence of these events. The carcinogen-DNA adduct (marker for initiation) has also been used in assessing dose-response relationships at much lower dose levels than those used in in vivo carcinogenicity studies (Neumann, 1983).

BIOCHEMICAL MARKERS

Carcinogenesis, as noted above, involves three major steps: initiation, promotion, and tumor development. Biochemical markers for these steps are in various stages of development and are potentially useful in exploring the modes of action of carcinogens and in facilitating early diagnosis of cancer. The following is a brief discussion of this rapidly expanding field; additional information and references are provided by Ketterer (1981). The clinical implications of markers of human cancer of various organs and systems are provided in a book edited by Sell and Wahren (1981).

Biochemical Markers of Initiation

Initiation is associated with covalent binding of electrophilic carcinogens or their active metabolites to DNA. The carcinogen-DNA adduct can be demonstrated and quantified with a radiolabeled carcinogen. Initiation can also be determined, without the administration of a radioactive carcinogen, by the use of radio-immunoassay. This procedure can therefore be applied to situations wherein human exposure to a particular carcinogen is suspected.

The covalent binding of a carcinogen to DNA is usually followed by DNA repair. The repair exhibits as unscheduled DNA synthesis and can be determined by the uptake of labeled thymidine. Additional information on this topic is given in Chapter 10.

Biochemical Marker of Promotion

Promotion has been most extensively studied in skin carcinogenesis. A variety of biochemical changes have been noted in initiated as well as normal cells on treatment with promoters, the most active of which is TPA (12-O-tetradecanoyl phorbol-13acetate). The changes include accumulation of plasminogen activator and increased prostaglandin synthesis. Their biologic significance is evidenced by the fact that antiproteases, which inhibit plasminogen activator, and anti-inflammatory agents, which inhibit prostaglandin synthesis, prevent mouse skin tumorigenesis promoted by TPA.

A liver tumor initiated by acetylaminofluorene (AAF) has been shown to be promoted by phenobarbital, DDT, polychlorinated biphenyls (PCB), and buty-lated hydroxytoluene (BHT). Certain enzymes (e.g., glucose-6-phosphatase and adenosine triphosphatase) are decreased, whereas others (e.g., γ-glutamyl trans-peptidase) are increased. These and other biochemical changes are being studied to determine their role as markers of preneoplasia in the liver.

Tumor Markers

α-Fetoprotein (AFP) is a product of fetal liver. It is often, although not always, produced by tumors of the testis and ovary. Nevertheless, it is a useful clinical tool. For example, AFP has been used to screen large populations for hepato-cellular carcinomas allowing early detection and treatment (Tang et al., 1980). Human chorionic gonadotropin (HCG) is a sensitive marker and can be used to detect cancer at a subclinical phase. Mammary carcinomas are often associated with abnormal levels of biochemical parameters such as carcinoembryonic antigen, ferritin, and C-reactive protein. Unfortunately, these changes generally appear only when the tumor has become metastatic, hence too late to be of value in the early diagnosis of cancer. Nevertheless, these are useful in evaluating the effect of clinical treatment and in following remissions and relapses, as shown by, for example, Fritsche (1982).

EVALUATION

Preliminary Assessment

A variety of information can be used in a preliminary evaluation of the carcinogenic potential of a chemical.

Chemical Structure A number of chemicals are known to be carcinogenic. A list of known and suspected human carcinogens is presented in Table 9-1. In addition, a large number of chemicals have been shown to be carcinogenic in animals (see "Genotoxic Carcinogens"). While chemicals have structures similar to any of these or other carcinogens/mutagens are not necessarily carcinogens, they should be assigned high priority in carcinogenicity testing programs.

Mutagenicity Mutagenic agents produce heritable genetic changes essentially through their effects on DNA. Thus their action is similar to that of genotoxic carcinogens. The mutagenicity tests also provide information on the mode of action as well as on the question as to whether metabolic activation is required for the mutagenicity.

Because each of the various mutagenicity tests may yield false-positive or false-negative results, it is advisable to carry out a proper combination of them. While positive results from these tests do not constitute positive evidence that the chemical is carcinogenic, they do indicate that extensive testing is required. On the other hand, negative results do not establish the safety of the chemical.

Limited Carcinogenicity Tests The endpoint in these tests is tumor formation. Therefore, certain chemicals, such as cocarcinogens that yield negative results in mutagenesis tests, may be positive in these tests. Positive results from more than one of these limited carcinogenicity tests may be considered unequivocal qualitative evidence of carcinogenicity.

It has been proposed (Bull and Rereira, 1982) that the carcinogenesis testing matrix be composed of the following mutagenesis and limited carcinogenesis tests: (1) mouse skin initiation/promotion, (2) strain A mouse lung adenoma, (3) rat liver foci, (4) cell transformation, and (5) in vivo sister chromatid exchange.

Definitive Assessment

Data from well-designed and properly executed long-term carcinogenicity studies generally provide a sound basis for assessment of the carcinogenic potential.

General Considerations Results from these studies are generally more reliable than those from the rapid screening tests. But the conclusiveness of the results depend on a number of factors. For example, too few animals surviving until tumor development may preclude statistical analysis of the data. This event may occur as a result of insufficient animals placed in each dosage group and/or excessive mortality resulting from improper husbandry or from competing toxicity of the chemical given at inordinately high dose levels.

The thoroughness of the postmortem examination also plays an important role. This applies to the gross as well as the microscopic examinations. Tumors in tissues and organs may be overlooked if they are subjected only to a cursory inspection. Special techniques may be required for proper examination of certain organs, e.g., the urinary bladder. Concomitant events such as stones and parasites in the bladder must be looked for and their presence or absence recorded. Proper fixation and staining of the tissues facilitate their microscopic examination.

Tumor Incidence As noted at the beginning of the chapter, carcinogenesis may manifest in one of the four forms or any combination thereof. An appreciable increase in the tumor-bearing animals is the most common form. The occurrence of unusual tumor is an important phenomenon if there are a significant number of them; when one or only a few of them are detected, further critical examination is required. Shortening of the latency period is readily noted with dermal and subcutaneous tumors. The latency of visceral tumor is, in practice, equivalent to the survival of the tumor-bearing animals because the tumor development is, in general, positively diagnosed only at autopsy. An increase in the number of tumors per animal without a concomitant increase in the tumor-bearing animals usually indicates cocarcinogenicity only.

As there remain doubts about the precise meaning of some of the terms used in describing tumors, descriptions of the morphology of the tumors and their relation with the surrounding tissues are desirable.

The tumors in the experimental animals may not be at the same stage of development. The stages may include, for example, atypical hyperplasia, benign tumors, carcinomas in situ, invasion of adjacent tissues, and metastasis to other parts of the body. Although tumors of the same type but at different stages should be separately tabulated, they should be combined for statistical analysis.

Dose-response Relationship As a rule, a positive dose-response relationship is apparent. However, there may be a lower tumor incidence in the high-dose group. This phenomenon usually results from poor survival among these animals, which succumb to competing toxic effects of the chemical.

Reproducibility of the Results The confidence in a carcinogenicity study is enhanced if the results are produced in another strain of animals. Reproducibility in another species is even more significant. However, if negative results are obtained in another species, this fact may not nullify the positive findings but does justify further investigation. For example, there may be differences in their biotransformation of the chemical or variations in the precise composition of the product used.

Evaluation of Safety/Risk

The various approaches used in the evaluation of the safety/risk of carcinogens are discussed in Chapter 7. The following points, however, appear worthy of reiterating.

First, while the tests enumerated above are a valuable basis for toxicologic evaluation, other data relating to the mechanism of action and influences of modifying factors, are also essential (Interdisciplinary Panel, 1984). The significant differences between genotoxic and epigenetic carcinogens as summarized in Table 9-1 are also considered as valid reasons for assessing their risks differently (see Williams, 1984).

Furthermore, there are chemicals with carcinogenicity secondary to non-carcinogenic biologic or physical effects that are elicited only at dose levels that could never be approached in realistic human exposure situations. There was general consensus that there are threshold doses for secondary carcinogens (Lu, 1976; Golberg, 1978).

Carcinogens also differ in the potency and latent periods. Some carcinogens are active in a particular species, whereas others affect several species and strains of animals. All these factors must be taken into account in evaluating the safety/risk of carcinogens.

Finally, it is important to bear in mind that chemicals differ tremendously in their value to humans. For example, a food color can normally be banned on the basis of suggestive carcinogenicity data. On the other hand, life-saving drugs, even when there is evidence of their carcinogenicity in humans may still be used clinically. There are also environmental carcinogens that cannot be eliminated with present technology.

REFERENCES

Berenblum, I., and Shubik, P. (1947) A new quantitative approach to the study of the stages of chemical carcinogenesis in the mouse's skin. *Br. J. Cancer* 1:383–391.

Berenblum, I., and Shubik, P. (1949) An experimental study of the initiating stage of carcinogenesis, and a re-examination of the somatic cell mutation theory of cancer. *Br. J. Cancer* 3:109–118.

Bull, R. J., and Pereira, M. A. (1982) Development of a short-term testing matrix for estimating relative carcinogenic risk. *J. Am. Coll. Toxicol.* 1:1–15.

Fritsche, H. A. (1982) Tumor marker tests in patient monitoring. *Lab. Med.* 13: 528–533.

Gehring, P. J., Watanabe, P. G., and Blau, G. E. (1979) Risk assessment of environmental carcinogens utilizing pharmacokinetic parameters. *Ann. NY Acad. Sci.* 329:137-152.

Golberg, L. (1978) Consideration of experimental thresholds. In: *Proceedings of the First International Congress on Toxicology*. Eds. G. L. Plaa and W. A. M. Duncan. New York: Academic Press.

Goldfarb, S., and Pugh, M. B. (1982) The origin and significance of hyperplastic hepatocellular islands and nodules in hepatic carcinogenesis. *J. Am. Coll. Toxicol.* 1:119-144.

Green, S., Collins, T. F. X., and Page, N. P. (1981) Special tests for mutagenicity, teratogenicity and carcinogenicity. In: *Toxicology: Principles and Practice, Vol. 1*. Ed. A. L. Reeves. New York: John Wiley.

Huggins, C., Briziarelli, G., and Sutton, H., Jr. (1959) Rapid induction of mammary carcinoma in the rat and the influence of hormones on the tumors. *J. Exp. Med.* 109:25-41.

IARC (1979) IARC Monographs, Suppl. 1. Chemicals and Industrial Processes Associated with Cancer in Humans. Lyons, France: International Agency for Research on Cancer.

IARC (1980a) *Basic requirements for long-term assays for carcinogenicity*. IARC Monographs, Suppl. 2, pp. 21-83. Lyons, France: International Agency for Research on Cancer.

IARC (1980b) *Rationale for deployment of short-term assays for evidence of carcinogenicity*. IARC Monographs, Suppl. 2, pp. 295-308. Lyons, France: International Agency for Research on Cancer.

International Commission for Protection against Environmental Mutagens and Carcinogens (1982) Mutagenesis testing as an approach to carcinogenesis. *Mutat. Res.* 99:73-91.

Interdisciplinary Panel on Carcinogenicity (1984) Criteria for evidence of chemical carcinogenicity. *Science* 225:682-687.

Ketterer, B. (1981) Biochemical markers in carcinogenesis. In: *Testing for Toxicity*. Ed. J. W. Gorrod. London: Taylor & Francis.

Kraybill, H. F. (1977) Conceptual approaches to the assessment of nonoccupational cancer. In: *Environmental Cancer*. Eds. H. F. Kraybill and M. A. Mehlman. Washington, D.C.: Hemisphere.

Lu, F. C. (1976) Threshold doses in chemical carcinogenesis: Introductory remarks. *Oncology* 33:50.

Neumann, H. G. (1983) The dose-response of DNA interactions of aminostilbene derivatives and other chemical carcinogens. In: *Developments in Science and Practice of Toxicology*. Eds. A. W. Hayes and T. S. Miya. New York: Eselvier Science.

OECD (1981) *OECD Guidelines for Testing of Chemicals*. Paris, France: Organization for Economic Cooperation and Development.

Page, N. P. (1977) Current concepts of a bioassay program in environmental carcinogenesis. In: *Environmental Cancer*. Eds. H. F. Kraybill and M. A. Mehlman. Washington, D.C.: Hemisphere.

Pereira, M. A. (1982) Mouse skin bioassay for chemical carcinogens. *J. Am. Coll. Toxicol.* 1:47-82.

Rashko, D., and Brand, G. (1983) Chromosomal aberrations in foreign body tumorigenesis of mice. *Proc. Soc. Exp. Biol. Med.* 172:382–388.

Sell, S., and Wahren, B. (1981) *Human Cancer Markers.* Clifton, N.J.: Humana.

Shimkin, M. B., and Stoner, G. D. (1975) Lung tumors in mice: Application to carcinogenesis bioassay. *Adv. Cancer Res.* 21:2–58.

Slaga, T. J., Fischer, S. M., Triplett, L. L., and Nesnow, S. (1982) Comparison of complete carcinogenesis and tumor initiation in mouse skin: Tumor initiation-promotion a reliable short-term assay. *J. Am. Coll. Toxicol.* 1:83–99.

Sunderman, F. W., Jr. (1984) Recent advances in metal carcinogenesis. *Ann. Clin. Lab. Sci.* 14:93–122.

Svoboda, D. J., and Reddy, J. K. (1975) Some effects of chemical carcinogens on cell organelles. In: *Cancer: A Comprehensive Treatise, Vol. 1.* Ed. F. F. Becker. New York: Plenum Press.

Tang, Z., Yang, B., Tang, C., Yu, Y., Lin, Z., and Weng, H. (1980) Evaluation of population screening for hepatocellular carcinoma. *Ch. Med. J.* 93:795–799.

Task Force (1982) Animal data in hazard evaluation: Paths and pitfalls. Task Force of Past Presidents of the Society of Toxicology. *Fundam. Appl. Toxicol.* 2:101–107.

Trosko, J. E., and Chang, C. C. (1983) Potential role of intercellular communication in the rate-limiting step in carcinogenesis. *J. Am. Coll. Toxicol.* 2(3):5–22.

Weinstein, I. B. (1980) Evaluating substances for promotion, cofactor effects and synergy in the carcinogenic process. *J. Environ. Pathol. Toxicol.* 3(4): 89–101.

Weisburger, J. H., and Williams, G. M. (1980) Chemical carcinogens. In: *Casarett and Doull's Toxicology.* Eds. J. Doull, Klaassen, and Amdur. New York: Macmillan.

Weisburger, J. H., and Williams, G. M. (1981) Basic requirements of health risk analysis: The decision point approach for systematic carcinogen testing. In: *Proceedings of the Third Life Sciences Symposium on Health Risk Analysis.* Philadelphia: Franklin Press.

WHO (1978) *Principles and Methods for Evaluating the Toxicity of Chemicals.* Part 1, Environmental Health Criteria 6. Geneva: World Health Organization.

Williams, G. M. (1981) Liver carcinogenesis: The role for some chemicals of an epigenetic mechanism of liver-tumor promotion involving modification of the cell membrane. *Food Cosmet. Toxicol.* 19:577–583.

Williams, G. M. (1984) Modulation of chemical carcinogenesis by xenobiotics. *Fundam. Appl. Toxicol.* 4:325–344.

Williams, D. J., and Parry, G. (1975) Endoplasmic membrane is a source and a target for chemically reactive metabolic intermediates. *Biochem. Soc. Trans.* 3:69–70.

Williams, G. M., and Watanabe, K. (1978) Quantitative kinetics of development of N-2-florenylacetanilide-induced altered (hyperplastic) hepatocellular foci resistant to iron accumulation and of their reversion of persistence following removal of carcinogen. *J. Nat. Cancer Inst.* 61:113–121.

Wright, A. S., Akintowa, D. A. A., and Wooder, M. F. (1977) Studies on the interactions of dieldrin with mammalian liver cells at the subcellular level. *Ecotoxicol. Environ. Safety* 1:7–16.

ADDITIONAL READINGS

NCI (1976) *Guidelines for Carcinogen Bioassay in Small Rodents.* DHEW Publication No. (NIH) 76-801. Bethesda, Md.: National Cancer Institute.

Schmahl, D., Thomas, C., and Auer, P. (1977) *Iatrogenic Carcinogenesis.* Berlin: Springer-Verlag.

WHO (1961) *Evaluation of the Carcinogenic Hazards of Food Additives.* WHO Tech. Rep. Ser. No. 220.

WHO (1969) *Principles for the Testing and Evaluation of Drugs for Carcinogenicity.* WHO Tech. Rep. Ser. 426.

Chapter 10

Mutagenesis

INTRODUCTION

Mutagenesis can occur as a result of interaction between mutagenic agents and the genetic materials of organisms. While spontaneous mutation and natural selection are the major means of evolution, a number of toxicants, in recent decades, have been found to be mutagenic.

Health Hazards

The eventual effects of human exposure to these mutagenic substances cannot be predicted at present. However, some of the spontaneous abortions, still-births, and heritable diseases have been shown to be related to changes in DNA molecules and to chromosomal aberrations. There are approximately 1000 dominant gene mutations responsible for various illnesses, including the heredi-tary neoplasms such as bilateral retinoblastoma, and about the same number of recessive gene disorders such as sickle-cell anemia, cystic fibrosis, and Tay-Sachs disease. In addition, chromosomal aberrations are associated with such diseases as Down's syndrome, Klinefelter's syndrome, and Turner's syndrome. These have been estimated to occur with an incidence of 0.5% among the live births in the United States. The true effects of any additional mutagen in the environment can only manifest after a lapse of several generations. The seriousness of this matter therefore warrants the extensive investigations in the various fields of mutagenesis.

A number of human diseases are the result of defects of the DNA repair systems. For example, patients with xeroderma pigmentosa are deficient in excision repair in the skin and the central nervous system; they are susceptible to ultraviolet light and many chemical carcinogens and thus are prone to developing skin tumors. Those with ataxia telangiectasia have such deficiencies in the lymphoid system and are known to be susceptible to X-rays and the carcinogen methyl nitronitrosoguanidine. Fanconi's anemia is associated with defective DNA repair in the blood and skeleton. The afflicted persons are susceptible to mitomycin C and psoralens. These and several other related diseases have been discussed by Cleaver (1980).

In addition, tests for mutagenicity in recent years have become more widely used because of their value as a rapid screening for carcinogenicity (see Chapter 9). This development stems mainly from the fact that most mutagens have been found to be carcinogens. Furthermore, these tests, with a variety of endpoints, are useful in the elaboration of the mode of action of carcinogens.

Categories of Mutagenesis Tests

It is well known that DNA, consisting of nucleotide bases, plays a key role in genetics. First, it transmits the genetic information from one generation of cells to the next through self-replication. This is done by the separation of the double strands of the DNA molecule and the synthesis of new daughter strands. Second, the genetic information coded in the DNA molecule is expressed through the transcription of a complementary RNA strand from one strand of DNA, which serves as a template, and the subsequent translation of the information from the RNA to the amino acids in proteins. Every set of three nucleotide bases, a codon, specifies an amino acid. Derangement of the bases therefore alters the amino acid content of the protein synthesized.

In earlier studies, the mutagenic activity was demonstrated mainly in fruit flies and onion root tips because of the simpler techniques involved. More recently, many new test systems have been developed. They range in complexity from microorganisms to intact mammals. The use of such widely different organisms is based on the fact that all double-stranded DNA share the same biochemical characteristics, which are listed in Table 10-1.

At present, there are more than 100 test systems. A number of exemplary tests are outlined in this chapter under four major categories, namely, gene mutation, chromosomal effects, DNA repair and recombination, and others.

Table 10-1 Basic Biochemical Characteristics of All Double-Stranded DNA

1. DNA consists of two different purines (guanine, adenine) and two different pyrimidines (thymine and cytosine).
2. A nucleotide pair consists of one purine and one pyrimidine [adenine/thymine (A-T) or guanine/cytosine (G-C)].
3. Nucleotide pairs are connected into a double helix molecule by sugar-phosphate backbone linkages and hydrogen bonding.
4. The A-T base pair is held by two hydrogen bonds, while the G-C is held by three.
5. The distance between each base pair in a molecule is 3.4 Å, producing 10 nucleotide pairs per turn of the DNA helix.
6. The number of adenine molecules must equal the number of thymine molecules in a DNA molecule. The same relationship exists for guanine and cytosine molecules. However, the ratio of A-T to G-C base pairs may vary in DNA from species to species.
7. The two strands of the double helix are complementary and antiparallel with respect to the polarity of the two sugar-phosphate backbones, one strand being 3'-5' and the other being 5'-3' with respect to the terminal OH group on the ribose sugar.
8. DNA replicates by a semiconservative method in which the two strands separate and each is used as a template for the synthesis of a new complementary strand.
9. The rate of DNA nucleotide polymerization during replication is approximately 600 nucleotides per second. The helix must unwind to form remplates at a rate of 3600 rpm to accommodate this replication rate.
10. The DNA content of cells is variable (1.8×10^9 daltons for *Escherichia coli* to 1.9×10^{11} daltons for human cells).

Source: Brusick, 1980, p. 13.

Because of the brevity of their description, at least one reference is cited for each test. Additional references and more details are given on these and other tests in a publication of IARC (1980). Detailed descriptions of most of these tests are given in the Guidelines of EPA (1982) and OECD (1983, 1984).

GENE MUTATION

Gene mutations involve additions or deletions of base pairs or substitution of a wrong base pair in the DNA molecules.

Substitutions consist of transitions and transversions. The former involves the replacement of a purine (adenine, guanine) by another or a pyrimidine (cytosine, thymine) by another. With transversion, a purine is replaced by a pyrimidine, or vice versa.

When the number of base pairs added or deleted is not a multiple of three, the amino acid sequence of the protein coded distal to the addition or deletion will be altered. This phenomenon is called frame-shift mutation and is likely to affect the biologic property of the protein. Figure 10-1 clearly illustrates the effects of a deletion and an addition of a nucleotide base.

In addition, a mutagen may be incorporated into the DNA molecule; it may also cause erroneous base pairing. These various changes in the DNA molecule may cause the substitution of a new amino acid in the subsequently coded protein molecule or result in a different sequence of amino acids in the protein synthesized. Furthermore, a protein synthesis termination codon may be formed, giving rise to a shortened protein. While the first type of effect may or may not result in a modification of the biologic property of the protein molecule, the latter two types almost invariably do.

Five basic tests are used for the detection of gene mutations.

Microbial Tests In Vitro

These involve prokaryotic and eukaryotic microorganisms.

Prokaryotic Microorganisms Such microorganisms consist of bacteria. For the detection of point mutations the commonly used bacteria are *Salmonella typhimurium* and *Escherichia coli*. Most bacterial systems are intended to detect

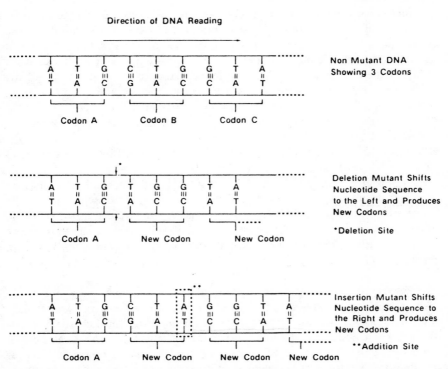

Figure 10-1 Frame-shift mutation resulting from deletion or insertion of a nucleotide base. A series of new codons is formed distal to the deletion or insertion, and hence new amino acids in the protein synthesized. (From Brusick, 1980, p. 28.)

reverse mutation. For example, the Ames test (Ames, 1971) measures the reversion of histidine-dependent mutants of *S. typhimurium* to the histidine-independent wild type. The mutants are incubated in a medium that contains insufficient histidine to permit visible growth. If the toxicant added to the culture medium is capable of inducing reverse mutation, then the bacteria can become histidine-independent and grow appreciably in the histidine-deficient medium. It is customary to use several strains because of their specificity. Their mutation to histidine-independency results from either frame-shift or base-pair substitution; different mutagens may affect one strain but not the other.

A number of strains of *S. typhimurium* have been rendered more sensitive to the effects of mutagens through alterations in the permeability of their cell walls (deficient in lipopolysaccharide) and in their DNA excision repair capabilities (through a specific deletion in the DNA molecule) and through the bearing of an ampicillin-resistance factor (Ames et al., 1975; McCann et al., 1975).

Since many mutagens are inactive before bioactivation, the test can be carried out with a bioactivating system included in the in vitro procedure. The bioactivating system usually consists of the microsomal fraction (containing the mixed-function oxidase system) of the liver of the rat or other animals, although the human liver is also used for special purposes. The activity of the microsomal enzyme is usually enhanced by pretreating the animal with an inducing agent, such as 3-methylcholanthrene, phenobarbital, or polychlorinated biphenyls (PCB). Appropriate cofactors are also added to the mixture prior to incubation (Ames et al., 1973). For such tests, the liquid suspension assay is better than the plate assay since bioactivation can proceed over a longer period of time.

Strains of *E. coli*, which are deficient in various degrees in DNA repair, are also used in mutagenesis tests. The wild type of *E. coli* can better survive the effect of a mutagen on DNA through normal repair mechanism, whereas the mutants cannot. Although most of the microbial systems are designed to detect reverse mutations, the *E. coli* strain of Mohn can detect forward mutations, e.g., resistance against 5-methyltryptophan (Mohn et al., 1974).

Eukaryotic Microorganisms Certain strains of *Saccharomyces, Schizosaccharomyces, Neurospora,* and *Aspergillus* have been developed to detect mainly reverse mutations and, to a limited extent, forward mutations. Like the bacterial systems, these systems in general also include bioactivating enzymes and cofactors. For example, a type of mutant of *Saccharomyces cerevisiae* requires adenine and produces red-pigmented colonies, whereas the while type microorganisms are adenine-independent and produce white colonies. Thus the reverse mutation can be determined by the prevalence of white colonies (Brusick and Mayer, 1973). A procedure using *Neurospora crassa* has been described by

De Serres and Malling (1971). The mutants form purple colonies, while the wild strain forms white colonies.

Microbial Tests In Vivo (Host-Mediated Assay)

In this type of test, the microorganisms are injected into the peritoneal cavity of the host mammal (usually the mouse). They can also be injected into the circulatory system or the testes. The toxicant is injected into the host, usually prior to the introduction of the microorganisms. After a few hours elapse, the host is sacrificed. The microorganisms are then collected and examined for manifestations of mutation. These assays have the advantage of incorporating the biotransformation of the toxicant in the host mammal but have the drawback that the microorganisms can only be kept in the host for a relatively short time. Apart from microorganisms, cells from multicellular animals can also be used in the host-mediated assay (Gabridge and Legator, 1969). Despite its theoretical advantage, the procedure has been found to be insensitive to certain types of carcinogens and hence is unsuitable as a routine screening procedure (Simmons, 1979).

A modified procedure involves pretreatment of the host with a toxicant, collecting the urine from the host, and injecting the urine, which may contain a high concentration of the metabolite(s) of the toxicant, back into the host. This modified procedure demonstrates positive mutagenicity with 2-acetylaminofluorene, which yields negative results with the regular host-mediated assay (Durston and Ames, 1974).

Insects

The fruit fly *Drosophila melanogaster* is the most commonly used insect. It is well characterized genetically. It has the advantage over microorganisms in that it metabolizes toxicants in a manner that is similar to mammals. Furthermore, it is superior to mammals in two respects, namely, its generation time is only 12-14 days, and it can be tested in sufficient numbers at much lower cost (Wurgler et al., 1977).

The sex-linked recessive lethal test measures the lethal effect on the F_2 males after exposing the males of the parental generation. It is the preferred procedure because the X chromosome represents about 20% of the total genome; hence it can respond to a variety of genetic effects, including point mutation and short deletions (Abrahamson and Lewis, 1971).

Mammalian Cells in Culture

The commonly used systems include cells from mouse lymphoma (Clive and Spector, 1975), human lymphoblasts (Sato et al., 1972), and cells from the lung, ovary, and other tissues of Chinese hamsters (Chu, 1971). These cells usually maintain a near-diploid chromosome number, grow actively, and have high cloning efficiency. Both forward and reverse mutations can occur, and the mutants responsd selectively to nutritional, biochemical, serologic, and drug-resistant growth manipulations.

For example, cells from mouse lymphoma, which are heterozygous at the thymidine kinase locus (TK+/−), may undergo forward mutation, e.g., via the action of a mutagen, and become TK−/−. Both genotype TK+/− and TK−/− can grow in normal medium, but TK−/− can also grow in a medium containing 5-bromo-2′-deoxyuridine (BrdU). The mutagenicity of a toxicant can thus be determined by comparing the growth of the lymphoma cells in the presence and absence of the toxicant both in a medium containing BrdU and in a normal medium.

In Chinese hamsters, as in humans, the use of preformed hypoxanthine and guanine is controlled by an X-linked gene. Mutant cells at these loci are deficient in the enzyme hypoxanthine-guanine phosphoribosyl transferase and can be identified by their resistance to toxic purine analogs, such as 8-azaguanine or 6-thioguanine, that kill the cells that utilize these analogs.

These cell lines are generally deficient in metabolizing enzymes. Therefore, such enzyme systems are often added (*microsome-mediated*). Alternatively, these cells can be cocultivated with other cells that possess greater ability to biotransform toxicants. Such a *cell-mediated* system was first described by Huberman and Sachs (1974). A new approach suggested by Williams (1979) involves the use of freshly isolated hepatocytes as a feeder system. It offers an additional advantage of having capabilities to conjugate as well as to degrade toxicants. In the *host-mediated* tests the target cells are inoculated into an animal that receives the chemical to be tested (Fischer et al., 1974).

Gene Mutation Tests in Mice

The Specific Locus Test   This was developed by Russell (1951) for determining the mutagenicity of ionizing radiation in the germ cells. This procedure was later adapted to assess the mutagenicity of chemicals (Searle, 1975). This test has the advantage of directly detecting in intact mammals the mutagenic effects of toxicants in the germ cells, but it usually requires a very large number of animals.

It involves exposing nonmutant mice to the chemical and subsequently mating them to a multiple-recessive stock. Mutant offspring have altered phenotypes expressed in hair color, hair structure, eye color, ear length, and other traits. Some mutants are mosaic rather than whole animal. Mutation can also be detected by the rejection or acceptance of skin grafts made between first-generation offspring. It can be further characterized immunogenetically (Bailey and Kohn, 1965). A variety of biochemical techniques have been used in detecting altered proteins produced by genetic changes (see IARC, 1980).

The Mouse Spot Test This test is designed to detect gene mutation in somatic cells. Basically it involves treating pregnant mice whose embryos are heterozygous at specific coat color loci and examining the newborn for any mosaic patches in the fur. Such patches indicate the formation of clones of mutant cells that are responsible for the color of the fur. This test is relatively inexpensive and takes only a few weeks to complete. Although it may yield false-positive results, it has not yet yielded false-negative results. The spot test is therefore a useful prescreen for heritable germinal mutations in mammals (Russell, 1978).

CHROMOSOMAL EFFECTS

The effect of a toxicant on chromosomes may manifest as structural aberrations or as changes in their number. The former include deletions, duplications, and translocations. The latter involves a decrease or increase in the number of the chromosomes. Some of the effects are heritable.

The mode of action underlying these effects may involve molecular cross-linkage, which may cause an arrest of the synthesis of DNA, thereby leaving a gap in the chromosome. An unsuccessful repair of the DNA damage may also be responsible. Nondisjunction (failure of a pair of chromosomes to separate during mitotic division) can lead to mosaicism. A nondisjunction during gametogenesis (meiotic nondisjunction) gives rise to daughter cells that contain either one extra chromosome or one less than normal. The former is known as *trisomy* and the latter *monosomy*.

A number of test systems have been developed to determine the chromosomal effects. The following are the major systems.

Insects

Drosophilia melanogastor has the advantage in that the chromosomes of some of its cells are superior in size and morphology. In addition, the chromosomal effects can be readily confirmed genetically, e.g., the sex-linked recessive lethality. The chromosomal effects include loss of X and Y chromosomes, and translocations of fragments between second and third chromosomes.

Effects on the sex chromosome can also be detected by phenotypic changes, e.g., body color and color and shape of the eye (National Research Council, 1983).

Cytogenetic Studies with Mammalian Cells

In Vitro Tests For cytogenetic tests, the commonly used cells are derived from mouse lymphoma, Chinese hamster ovaries, and human lymphocytes. These cells are cultured in suitable media. They are then exposed to different concentrations of the test chemical in the presence or absence of a bioactivator system (usually the microsomal fraction of the rat liver homogenate). The test generally includes two positive control mutagens, namely, ethylmethane sulfonate, which is direct-acting, and dimethylnitrosamine, which requires bioactivation. After an appropriate incubation period, the cell division is arrested by the addition of colchicine. The cells are then mounted, stained, and scored (Cohen and Hierschhorn, 1971).

An example of scoring of aberrations is shown below. Definitions of these terms are provided by Brusick (1980): chromatid gap, chromatid break, chromosome gap, chromatid deletion, fragment, acentric fragment, translocation, triradial, quadriradial, pulverized chromosome, pulverized chromosomes, pulverized cells, ring chromosome, dicentric chromosome, minute chromosome, greater than 10 aberrations, polypoid, hyperploid.

In Vivo Tests Mammalian cells used in the in vivo study of chromosomal effects include germ cells and somatic tissues. The chemical to be tested is administered to intact animals, such as rodents (mice, rats, hamsters) and humans. The somatic tissues commonly used are bone marrow and peripheral lymphocytes. A classic protocol using bone marrow from mice, rats, or hamsters has been provided by the Ad Hoc Committee of the Environmental Mutagen Society and the Institute for Medical Research (1972). The scoring is the same as in the in vitro test.

A somewhat simpler in vivo procedure is the *micronucleus* test. It involves the use of polychromatic erythrocyte stem cells of CD-1 mice. Six hours after two treatments with the test chemical, given 24 hours apart, the animals are killed and the bone marrow is collected from both femurs. An increase in micronucleated cells over the controls (about 0.5%) is considered positive (Schmid, 1976). These micronuclei represent fragments of chromosome and chromatid resulting from spindle/centromere dysfunction.

For tests on *germ cells*, the male animals is usually used. In order to allow cells of different stages of spermatogenesis to be exposed, the chemical is given daily for 5 days and the animals sacrificed 1, 3, and 5 weeks following the last dose. The sperm is collected surgically from the caudae epididymides. The incidence of abnormal spermheads is determined, after mounting and staining, and it is compared with the negative and positive controls (Wyrobek and Bruce, 1975).

Dominant Lethal Test in Rodents

This test is designed to demonstrate toxic effects on germ cells in the intact male animal, usually the mouse or rat. The effects can manifest in the mated females as dead implantations and/or preimplantation losses (the difference between the number of corpora lutea and the number of implantations). These effects are generally due to chromosomal damages, which lead to developmental errors that are fatal to the zygote. However, other cytotoxic effects can also cause early fetal death. Specific protocols have been provided in a number of published articles (Ehling et al., 1978).

Heritable Translocation Test in Mice

This test is intended to detect the heritability of chromosomal damages. The damages, consisting of reciprocal translocation in the germ line cells of the treated male mice, are transmitted to the offspring. By mating the male F_1 progeny with untreated female mice, the chromosomal effects are revealed by a reduction of viable fetuses. The presence of these reciprocal translocations can be verified by the presence of translocation figures among the double tetrads at meiosis (Generoso et al., 1978; Adler, 1980).

DNA REPAIR AND RECOMBINATION

These biologic processes are not mutations per se, but they occur after DNA damage. These phenomena therefore indicate existence of DNA damages, which are caused essentially by mutagens.

Bacteria

Among *E. coli* there are those with normal DNA polymerase I enzyme, which is capable of repairing DNA damage, and those deficient in this enzyme. Mutagens induce DNA damage and thereby impair the growth of the *E. coli* that is deficient in the repair enzyme, whereas the growth of those with this enzyme is not affected. The DNA repair-efficient strain is included to rule out the effect of cytotoxicity (Rosenkranz et al., 1976; Slater et al., 1971).

Similarly, there are also recombination efficient and deficient strains of *Bacillus subtilis*. Damage to DNA is repaired in the former strain through recombination but not in the latter. Mutagens will thus inhibit the growth of the latter but not the former (Kada et al., 1972).

Yeasts

Various eukaryotic microorganisms, such as *Saccharomyces cerevisiae*, have been used to test the mutagenicity of chemicals by the induced mitotic crossing-over, mitotic gene conversion and reverse mutation (Zimmerman et al., 1975).

Mammalian Cells

Unscheduled DNA synthesis, an indication of DNA repair, can be detected in human cells in culture. The synthesis is determined by the amount of radioactive thymidine incorporated per unit weight of DNA over the control value. This is done both in the presence and absence of an added activator system (Stich and Laishes, 1973).

Such synthesis can also be determined in primary rat liver cells. The extent of DNA synthesis is determined using an autoradiographic method. Since these cells have sufficient metabolic activity, there is no need to add an activator system (Williams, 1977).

Sister Chromatid Exchange

This test measures reciprocal exchange of segments at homologous loci between sister chromatids, and can be done with mouse lymphoma cells, Chinese hamster ovary cells, and human lymphocytes. It basically involves labeling of cells with 5-BrdU. After two cycles of replication, the cells are stained with a fluorescent-plus-Giemsa technique. The frequency of sister chromatid exchanges per cell and per chromosome is scored and compared. The exchange is visible because in one chromatid the semiconservative replication of DNA results in a substitution of BrdU in *one* polynucleotide strand, and in the other chromatid the BrdU is substituted in *both* polynucleotide strands (Wolff, 1977).

OTHER TESTS

As noted in Chapter 9, a number of related tests are used to determine carcinogenicity.

In Vitro Transformation of Mouse Cells

Cells from the BALB/3T3 mouse are commonly used in this test. Others include Syrian hamster embryo cells, mouse 10T1/2 cells, and human cells. For references see Brusick (1980). Normally these cells will grow in the culture medium to form a monolayer. Those treated with a carcinogen, however, will reproduce without being attached to a solid surface and grow over the monolayer. The appearance of such multilayered colonies indicates malignant transformation. This endpoint can be confirmed by injecting these cells into syngeneic animals. In general, malignant tumors will develop if the cells have undergone transformation (Kakunaga, 1973). Therefore, in general, positive results from this test are especially significant.

Nuclear Enlargement Test

HeLa cells are grown in culture medium and treated with different concentrations of the chemical on test. After an appropriate duration, the cells are harvested and counted. They are then stripped of their cytoplasmic material and the size of the nucleus is determined with a particle counter. An increase in the nuclear size indicates carcinogenicity of the chemical (Finch et al., 1980).

EVALUATION

Need for Mutagenesis Studies

There is little doubt about the seriousness of mutagenesis. As stated earlier, many hereditary diseases are apparently associated with chromosomal aberrations, and dominant and recessive gene mutations. In addition, mutagenesis may contribute to the etiology of such common diseases as diabetes mellitus, epilepsy, schizophrenia, essential hypertension, cataracts, aging, and heart disease. Finally, the close relationship between mutagens and carcinogens must be borne in mind.

Thus, there is an enormous challenge to the toxicologist in identifying the mutagens to which humans are exposed and in defining their risks. So far, achievement in this area has been limited. This state of affairs stems mainly from the fact that this special discipline of toxicology has had only a very brief history. New test systems are still being developed, and the validity and limitations of the existing tests are still being studied. Nevertheless, the current knowledge in this field does provide a basis for a rational approach to the screening of toxicants for their mutagenic/carcinogenic potential.

Criteria for Selecting Substances for Testing

In view of the enormous number of natural and man-made substances to which humans are exposed, and the large number of mutagenesis tests that are available, it is not feasible to carry out all tests on all substances. There is, therefore, a need to establish criteria for selecting substances to be tested and the types of tests to be conducted. The criteria for selecting drugs have been considered by a WHO scientific group (WHO, 1971). These may be restated as follows to cover drugs and other substances:

1 Substances that are chemically, pharmacologically, and biochemically related to known or suspected mutagens
2 Substances that exhibit certain toxic effects in animals, such as depression of bone marrow, inhibition of spermatogenesis or oogenesis, inhibition of mitosis (e.g., in intestinal epithelium), teratogenicity, causation of sterility or semisterility in reproduction studies, and inhibition of immune response
3 Substances to which humans are exposed for a long duration
4 Substances to which a large proportion of the population is exposed

Selection of Test Systems

Since mutagens affect the genetic material in different ways, they may yield negative results in one test although positive in others. To rule out false-negatives (and false-positives), it is advisable to conduct several tests, preferably of different categories.

The U.S. Environmental Protection Agency (EPA, 1978) proposed that a battery of eight different kinds of tests be conducted.

1   For detecting gene mutation, a minimum of three tests be selected from these: (1) bacteria, (2) yeasts, (3) insects (e.g., sex-linked recessive lethal test), (4) mammalian somatic cells in culture, and (5) the mouse specific locus test

2   For detecting chromosomal aberrations, a minimum of three tests be selected from these: (1) in vivo cytogenetic tests in mammals, (2) tests insects for heritable chromosomal effects, (3) dominant lethal effect in rodents, and (4) heritable translocation tests in rats

3   For detecting primary DNA damage, a minimum of two tests be selected from these: (1) DNA repair in bacteria, (2) unscheduled DNA repair synthesis in mammalian cells, (3) mitotic recombination and/or gene conversion in yeast, and (4) sister chromatid exchange. Where applicable, these should be conducted with and without metabolic activation.

There is a wide range in the cost and time required for various test systems. The in vitro microbial tests with or without activation are inexpensive and can be conducted in a short time. In the other extreme, the in vivo specific locus mutation tests in mammals are very costly and time-consuming.

In practice, a tier system of testing is adopted. It starts with certain microbial tests and progresses through insects, mammalian cells in culture, cytogenetic tests in vivo, the spot test in mice, to specific locus test in mammals (Epler et al., 1978).

A more recent document of EPA (1982) provides detailed descriptions of the above-mentioned tests as well as those of the following:

Chromosomal Effects

In vivo mammalian cytogenetics and chromosomal analysis
In vivo micronucleus assay

DNA Effects

In vivo sister chromatid exchange assay

OECD (1983), 1984) also published guidelines on seven mutagenesis tests:

Salmonella typhimurium reverse mutation assay
E. coli reverse mutation assay
In vitro mammalian cytogenetic test
In vivo mammalian bone marrow cytogenetic test—chromosomal analysis
In vitro mammalian cell gene mutation tests
Micronucleus test
Sex-linked recessive lethal test in Drosophila melanogaster

The Committee on Chemical Environmental Mutagens of the National Research Council recommended a mutagen assessment program (National Research Council, 1983). It suggests that the mutagenesis tests be placed in three tiers. Tier I consists of (1) the *Salmonella*/microsome gene-mutation test, (2) a mammalian cell gene-mutation test, and (3) a mammalian cell chromosomal breakage test. If all tests are negative, the chemical is considered a presumed mammalian nonmutagen. If two of these tests are positive, it is classified as a presumed mammalian mutagen. If only one is positive, then the Tier II test (*Drosophila* sex-linked lethal-mutation) is conducted. For further screening of the most crucial chemicals, supplemental tests are done. A specific-locus test is recommended for chemicals with a potential mutagenicity in mammalian germ cells, and a dominant lethal test should be done for those having chromosomal effects.

It further suggests that (1) a large number of chemicals be screened with short-term tests, (2) the chemicals be classified according to their potency (their effective concentration), (3) one consider also the available carcinogenicity data, (4) test chemicals of crucial importance in mice, and (5) estimate their risks for humans.

Significance of Results

Relation Between Mutagenicity and Carcinogenicity   A number of investigators (e.g., Frohberg, 1973) have shown the relation between carcinogens and mutagens. More recently, McCann et al. (1975) reported on their study of 300 substances for mutagenicity in the *Salmonella*/microsome test. The results were compared with the reported carcinogenicity or noncarcinogenicity of these substances. The authors demonstrated a high correlation between these toxic effects: 90% (156/175) of carcinogens are mutagenic in the test. Few noncarcinogens showed any degree of mutagenicity.

Of the 18 carcinogens that yielded false-negative results, some have been shown to require other metabolic activation (e.g., cycasin and 1,2-dimethylhydrazine are not carcinogenic in germ-free animals, indicating the need for activation by intestinal flora). Others such as aminotriazole, thioacetamide, and thiourea are goitrogenic and cause thyroid tumors via a nonmutagenic mechanism (see also Chapter 9). Still others, e.g., auramine, are carcinogenic only because of their impurities. The mutagenicity of diethylstilbestrol could not be properly tested in this system because of its toxicity to the bacteria.

Validation studies have also been done on many other mutagenesis tests. The IARC publication (1980) includes the results of a large number of such studies, indicating different degrees of predictive value.

Heritable Effects   At present there is no direct correlation between laboratory tests for heritable mutations and human experience. Nevertheless, if a substance has been shown to be mutagenic in a variety of test systems including heritable mutations in intact mammals, it must be considered as a mutagen in humans unless there is convincing evidence to the contrary. Furthermore, for many chemicals, e.g., food additives, pesticides, cosmetics, and most drugs, where human exposure can be avoided, much less information will be sufficient to warrant suspension of their use (see Flamm, 1977). At present no reliable method is available for estimating risks associated with mutagens by their strength (National Research Council, 1983).

As mentioned above, the study of mutagenesis is a new discipline. The rapidly accumulating knowledge in this field will, in all probability, affect the interpretation of the significance of the mutagenicity testing results as well as the selection of the test systems for screening toxicants.

REFERENCES

Abrahamson, S., and Lewis, E. B. (1971) The detection of mutagens in *Drosophila melanogaster*. In: *Chemical Mutagens: Principles and Methods for Their Detection*, Vol. 2, pp. 461–487. Ed. A. Hollander. New York: Plenum Press.

Ad Hoc Committee of the Environmental Mutagen Society and the Institute of Medical Research (1972) Chromosome methodologies in mutagen testing. *Toxicol. Appl. Pharmacol.* 22:269–275.

Adler, I. D. (1980) New approaches to mutagenicity studies in animals for carcinogenic and mutagenic agents. I. Modification of heritable translocation test. *Teratog. Carcin. Mutagen.* 1:75–86.

Ames, B. N. (1971) The detection of chemical mutagens with enteric bacteria. In: *Chemical Mutagens: Principles and Methods for Their Detection*, Vol. 1, pp. 267–282. Ed. A. Hollander. New York: Plenum Press.

Ames, B. N., Durston, W. E., Yamasaki, E., and Lee, F. D. (1973) Carcinogens are mutagens: A simple test system combining liver homogenates for activation and bacteria for detection. *Proc. Nat. Acad. Sci. (USA)* 70:2281–2285.

Ames, B. N., McCann, J., and Yamasaki, E. (1975) Methods for detecting carcinogens and mutagens with the *Salmonella*/mammalian-microsome mutagenicity test. *Mutat. Res.* 31:347–364.

Bailey, D. W., and Kohn, H. I. (1965) Inherited histocompatibility changes in progeny of irradiated and unirradiated inbred mice. *Genet. Res.* 6:330–340.

Brusick, D. J. (1980) *Principles of Genetic Toxicology*. New York: Plenum Press.

Brusick, D. J., and Mayer, V. W. (1973) New developments in mutagenicity screening techniques with yeast. *Environ. Health Perspect.* 6:83–96.

Chu, E. H. Y. (1971) Induction and analysis of gene mutations in mammalian cells in culture. In: *Chemical Mutagens: Principles and Methods for Their Detection*, Vol. 2, pp. 441–444. Ed. A. Hollander. New York: Plenum Press.

Cleaver, J. E. (1980) DNA damage, repair systems and human hypersensitive diseases. *J. Environ. Pathol. Toxicol.* 3(4):53–68.

Clive, D., and Spector, J. F. S. (1975) Laboratory procedures for assessing specific locus mutations at the TK locus in cultured L5178Y mouse lymphoma cells. *Mutat. Res.* 31:17–29.

Cohen, M. M., and Hirschhorn, K. (1971) Cytogenetic studies in animals. In: *Chemical Mutagens: Principles and Methods for Their Detection*, Vol. 2, pp. 515–534. Ed. A. Hollander. New York: Plenum Press.

De Serres, F. J., and Malling, H. V. (1971) Measurement of recessive lethal damage over the entire genome and at two specific loci and the ad-3 region of a two-component heterokaryon of *Neurospora crassa*. In: *Chemical Mutagens: Principles and Methods for Their Detection*, Vol. 2, pp. 311–342. Ed. A. Hollander. New York: Plenum Press.

Durston, W. E., and Ames, B. N. (1974) Simple method for the detection of mutagens in urine: Studies with the carcinogen 2-acetylaminofluorene. *Proc. Nat. Acad. Sci. (USA)* 71:737–741.

Ehling, U. H., et al. (a work group set up by the group "Dominant Lethal Mutations of the Ad Hoc Committee on Chemogenetics") (1978) Standard protocol for the dominant lethal test on male mice. *Arch. Toxicol.* 39:173–185.

EPA (1978) Mutagenicity Testing in Pesticide Programs. *Fed. Reg.* 40(163), pp. 37388–37394.

EPA (1982) *Health Effects Test Guidelines*. Washington, D.C.: U.S. Environmental Protection Agency.

Epler, J. L., Larimer, F. W., Rao, T. K., Nix, C. E., and Ho, T. (1978) Energy-related pollutants in the environment: Use of short-term tests for mutagenicity in the isolation and identification of biohazards. *Environ. Health Perspect.* 27:11–20.

Finch, R. A., Evans, I. M., and Bosmann, H. B. (1980) Chemical carcinogen in vitro testing: A method for sizing cell nuclei in the nuclear enlargement assay. *Toxicol.* 15:145–154.

Fischer, G. A., Lee, S. Y., and Calabresi, P. (1974) Detection of chemical mutagens using a host-mediated assay (L5178Y) mutagenesis system. *Mutat. Res.* 26:501–511.

Flamm, W. G. (Chairman, DHEW Working Group on Mutagenicity Testing) (1977) Approaches to determining the mutagenic properties of chemicals: Risk to future generations. *J. Environ. Pathol. Toxicol.* 1:301–352.

Frohberg, H. (1973) Problems encountered in the toxicological testing of environmental chemicals. In: *Global Aspects of Chemistry, Toxicology as Applied to the Environment*. Eds. F. Coulston and F. Korte. New York: Academic Press.

Gabridge, M. G., and Legator, M. S. (1969) A host-mediated microbial assay for the detection of mutagenic compounds. *Proc. Soc. Exp. Biol. Med.* 130:831–834.

Generoso, W. M., Cain, K. T., and Huff, S. W. (1978) Inducibility by chemical mutagens of heritable translocations in male and female germ cells in mice. *Adv. Mod. Toxicol.* 5:109–129.

Huberman, E., and Sachs, L. (1974) Cell-mediated mutagenesis of mammalian cells with chemical carcinogens. *Int. J. Cancer* 13:326–333.

IARC (1980). *Long-Term and Short-Term Screening Assays for Carcinogens: A Critical Appraisal*. IARC Monographs, Suppl. 2. Lyon, France: International Agency for Research on Cancer.

Kada, T., Tutikawa, K., and Sadaie, Y. (1972) In vitro and host-mediated rec-assay procedures for screening chemical mutagens. *Mutat. Res.* 16:165–174.

Kakunaga, T. (1973) A quantitative system for assay of malignant transformation by chemical carcinogens using a clone derived from BALB/3T3. *Int. J. Cancer* 12:463–473.

Kilby, B. J., Legator, M., Nichols, W., and Ramel, C. (1984) *Handbook of Mutagenicity Test Procedures.* Amsterdam: Elsevier.

McCann, J., Choi, E., Yamasaki, E., and Ames, B. N. (1975) Detection of carcinogens as mutagens in the *Salmonella*/microsome tests assay of 300 chemicals. *Proc. Nat. Acad. Sci. (USA)* 72:5135–5139.

Mohn, G., Ellenberger, J., and McGregor, D. (1974) Development of mutagenicity tests using *E. coli* K12 as indicator organism. *Mutat. Res.* 25:187–196.

National Research Council (NRC) (1983) *Identifying and Estimating the Genetic Impact of Chemical Mutagens.* A report of the Committee on Chemical Environmental Mutagens, National Research Council. Washington, D.C.: National Academy Press.

OECD (Organization for Economic Cooperation and Development) (1983, 1984) *OECD Guidelines for Testing Chemicals.* Washington, D.C.: OECD Publications and Information Center.

Rosenkranz, H. S., Gutter, G., and Spek, W. J. (1976) Mutagenicity and DNA-modifying activity: A comparison of two microbial assays. *Mutat. Res.* 41:61–70.

Russell, L. B. (1978) Somatic Cells as indicators of germinal mutations in the mouse. *Environ. Health Perspect.* 24:113–116.

Russell, W. L. (1951) X-ray-induced mutations in mice. *Cold Spring Harbor Symp. Quant. Biol.* 16:327–336.

Sato, K., Slesinski, R. S., and Littlefield, J. W. (1972) Chemical mutagenesis at the phosphoribosyltransferase locus in cultured human lymphoblasts. *Proc. Nat. Acad. Sci. (USA)* 69:1246–1248.

Schmid, W. (1976) The micronucleus test. *Mutat. Res.* 31:9–15.

Searle, A. G. (1975) The specific locus test in the mouse. *Mutat. Res.* 31:277–290.

Simmons, V. F. (1979) In vitro mutagenicity assays of chemical carcinogens with *Salmonella typhimurium. J. Nat. Cancer Inst.* 62:893–899.

Slater, E. E., Anderson, M. D., and Rosenkranz, H. S. (1971) Rapid detection of mutagens and carcinogens. *Cancer Res.* 31:970–973.

Stich, H. F., and Laishes, B. A. (1973) DNA repair and chemical carcinogens. *Pathobiol. Annu.* 3:341–376.

WHO (1971) *The Evaluation of Testing of Drugs for Mutagenicity.* WHO Tech. Rep. Ser. 482. Geneva: World Health Organization.

Williams, G. M. (1977) The detection of chemical carcinogens by unscheduled DNA synthesis in rat liver primary cell culture. *Cancer Res.* 37:1845–1851.

Williams, G. M. (1979) The status of in vitro test systems utilizing DNA damage and repair for the screening of chemical carcinogens. *J. Assoc. Off. Anal. Chem.* 63:857–863.

Wolff, S. (1977) Sister chromatid exchange. *Ann. Rev. Genet.* 11:183–201.

Wurgler, F. E., Sobel, F. H., and Vogel, E. (1977) *Drosophila* as an assay system for detecting genetic changes. In: *Handbook of Mutagenicity Test Procedures.* Eds. B. J. Kilby, M. Legator, W. Nichols, and C. Ramel. Amsterdam: Elsevier/North Holland.

Wyrobek, A. J., and Bruce, W. R. (1975) Chemical induction of sperm abnormalities in mice. *Proc. Nat. Acad. Sci. (USA)* 72:4425–4429.

Zimmermann, F. K., Kern, R., and Rasenberger, A. (1975) A yeast strain for simultaneous detection of induced mitotic crossing over, mitotic gene conversion and reverse mutation. *Mutat. Res.* 28:381–388.

Chapter 11

Teratogenesis

INTRODUCTION

Historical Background

Teratogenesis is the formation of congenital defects. This type of illness has been known for decades and is an important cause of morbidity and mortality among newborns. For example, Murphy (1928) reviewed 320 human pregnancies and found 14 cases of children with small head circumference and mental retardation. Their mothers had been exposed to therapeutic radiation early in the pregnancy. Hale (1933) reported anophthalmia in the offspring of a sow deprived of vitamin A before pregnancy and during the first month of gestation. Warkany and Schraffenberger (1944) reported malformations resulting from nutritional deficiencies. Gregg (1941) suggested a relationship between the exposure of pregnant women to German measles and the blindness, deafness, and death among their offspring.

A connection was not suspected to exist between congenital malformation and chemicals because there was a tendency among toxicologists to assume that the natural protective mechanisms, e.g., detoxication, elimination, and placental barrier, were sufficient to shield the embryo from maternal exposure to chemicals. On the other hand, it was not unexpected that the natural protective mechanisms were ineffective against ionizing radiation, viruses, and nutritional deficiencies.

A new era in teratology was initiated as a result of the clinical use of thalidomide, a sedative-hypnotic. This drug, first introduced in the late 1950s in Germany, was found to be relatively nontoxic in experimental animals and in humans. Thus, while the therapeutic dose was 100 mg, ingestion of 14,000 mg by a person, with suicidal intent, did not result in death. It was used, among other indications, for the relief of morning sickness. In 1960, a few cases of phocomelia were reported. In the following year, there were many more cases. Phocomelia is a very rare type of congenital malformation, with shortening or absence of limbs. The causative agent in these cases was soon traced to the ingestion of thalidomide by the mothers, mainly between the third and eighth week of pregnancy. The use of the drug was promptly prohibited. In spite of that action, about 10,000 such malformed babies were born in a number of countries (Lenz and Knapp, 1962; Lenz, 1964). Because of the severity of the defects, elaborate prostheses were designed and utilized and special rehabilitation programs were instituted. Nevertheless, the profound, tragic effect on the malformed individuals and the traumatic impact on the families and society were so great that all feasible steps were instituted in an attempt to prevent the occurrence of such a man-made teratogenesis. One of these steps was to subject numerous drugs, food additives, pesticides, environmental contaminants and other chemicals to various types of testing to determine their potential teratogenicity.

Embryology

After fertilization, the ovum undergoes a precise sequence of cell proliferation, differentiation, migration, and organogenesis. The embryo then passes through a set of metamorphosis and a period of fetal development before birth.

Predifferentiation Stage During this stage the embryo is not susceptible to teratogenic agents. These agents either cause death of the embryo by killing all or most of the cells, or have no apparent effect on the embryo. Even when some mildly harmful effects have been produced, the surviving cells can compensate and form a normal embryo. This resistant stage varies from 5–9 days depending on the species.

Embryonic Stage This is the period when the cells undergo intensive differentiation, mobilization, and organization. It is during this period that most of the organogenesis takes place (Fig. 11-1). As a result, the embryo is most susceptible to the effects of teratogens. This period generally ends some time from

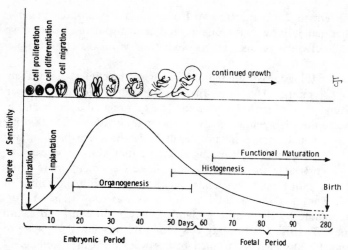

Figure 11-1 Stages of embryogenesis. After fertilization, the ovum undergoes cell proliferation, differentiation, and migration. These stages are followed by organogenesis, histogenesis, and functional maturation. The periods in days refer to human pregnancies; however, other mammals have essentially the same stages. (From Timbrell, 1982; Artwork: C. J. Timbrell.)

the 10th to the 14th day in rodents and in the 14th week of the gestation period in humans. Furthermore, not all organs are susceptible at the same time of the pregnancy. Figure 11-2 shows that the rat embryo is most susceptible between days 8 and 12 for most organs, but the palate and urogenital organs are more susceptible at a later stage.

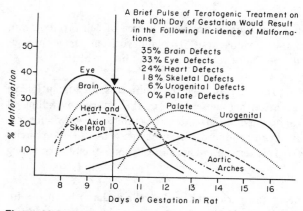

Figure 11-2 Expected incidences of malformation of different organs and systems the susceptibilities of which vary according to the days of gestation. A brief exposure to a teratogen on the 10th day of gestation is expected to induce a variety of malformations, with their incidences shown here. (Reprinted from *Teratology: Principles and Techniques*, by J. G. Wilson; by permission of the University of Chicago Press.)

Fetal Stage This stage is characterized by growth and functional maturation. Teratogens are thus unlikely to cause morphologic defects during this stage, but they may induce functional abnormalities. Whereas morphologic defects are in general readily detected at birth or shortly thereafter, functional abnormalities, e.g., CNS deficiencies, may not be diagnosed for some time after birth.

MODE OF ACTION OF TERATOGENS

A variety of chemicals have been shown to be teratogenic in animal models. A compilation of such chemicals is provided in Appendix 11-1. In view of the great diversity of the properties of these agents, it is not surprising that many different mechanisms are involved in their teratogenic effects.

Interference with Nucleic Acids

Numerous agents interfere with nucleic acid replication, transcription, or RNA translation. These include alkylating agents, antimetabolites, intercalating agents, and amino acid antagonists. Some of these chemicals per se are active; others require bioactivation, such as aflatoxin and thalidomide. Although some chemicals, e.g., carbon tetrachloride and nitrosamines, also yield reactive metabolites, their reactive metabolites are too unstable to reach the embryo. Therefore, these toxicants are not potent teratogens.

Deficiency of Energy Supply and Osmolarity

Certain teratogens can affect the energy supply for the metabolism of the organism by restricting the availability of substrates either directly (e.g., dietary deficiencies) or through the presence of analogs or antagonists of vitamins, essential amino acids, and others. In addition, hypoxia and agents inducing hypoxia (CO, CO_2) can be teratogenic by depriving the metabolic process of the required oxygen and probably also by the production of osmolar imbalances. These can induce edema and hematomas, which in turn can cause mechanical distortion and tissue ischemia.

Inhibition of Enzymes

Inhibitors of enzymes, e.g., 5-fluorouracil, can induce malformation through interference with differentiation or growth, by inhibiting thymidylate synthetase. Other examples include 6-aminonicotinamide, which inhibits glucose-6-phosphate dehydrogenase, and folate antagonists, which inhibit dihydrofolate reductase.

Others

Hypervitaminosis A may be associated with ultrastructural damage to cellular membranes in rodent embryos, a mechanism that may explain the teratogenicity of vitamin A. Physical agents that can cause malformations include radiation, hypothermia and hyperthermia, and mechanical trauma.

It should be noted that the mode of action of many teratogens is as yet uncertain. Furthermore, a potential teratogen may or may not exert teratogenic effects depending on such factors as bioactivating mechanism, stability of the reactive metabolites, ability to cross the placental barrier, and detoxifying capability of the embryonic tissues. Appropriate experimental testing for the teratogenicity of toxicants is therefore essential.

A comprehensive catalog of teratogens has been published (Shepard, 1980); Appendix 11-1 provides an abbreviated compilation.

TESTING PROCEDURES

Animals

Rats, rabbits, mice, and hamsters are the commonly used animals, because of their ready availability, easy handling, large litter size, and short gestational period. Pigs are sometimes used because they are phylogenetically more similar to humans and because their diet, unlike that of rabbits, is more similar to that of humans. WHO (1967) suggested the use of nonhuman primates because of their phylogenetic proximity to humans. Other animals such as dogs and cats have also been used by some investigators. The relative advantages and disadvantages of various species of animals for use in teratology have been described (Health and Welfare, Canada, 1973; Collins and Collins, 1976).

Because of the simplicity of the technique, the developing chick embryo had been widely used in the 1960s. However, it is now generally accepted that this model yields too many false-positives associated with its lack of a placenta and its susceptibility to such nonspecific factors as pH, specific gravity, and osmotic pressure.

The animals should be young, mature, and healthy. *Prima gravida* females are preferred.

With rats, at least 20 females are placed in each dose group; with rabbits, 12 females are used per dose (EPA, 1982). Smaller numbers of large animals such as dogs and nonhuman primates are used.

Administration of the Chemical

Dosage At least three dosage levels are used. The higher dosage should include some maternal (and/or fetal) toxicity, such as reduction in body weight. The lowest dosage should induce no observable ill effect. One or more doses should be appropriately interspersed between the two extremes.

In addition, two control groups are included. One of these is given the vehicle or physiologic saline, and the other receives a substance of known teratogenic activity. These groups will provide information on the incidence of *spontaneous* malformations and the sensitivity of the specific lot of animals under the existing experimental conditions. In addition to these contemporary controls, data from historical controls are also useful.

Route and Timing   The test substances should be administered by the route that simulates the human exposure situations. For food additives and contaminants, the chemical is preferably incorporated in the animal feeds. Oral drugs are generally administered by gastric gavage.

The timing of administering the chemical is important, as illustrated by the experiment of Tuchmann-Duplessis (1965) with 6-mercaptopurine, which produced either nervous and ocular defects or skeletal anomalies, depending on the timing. However, for routine teratologic studies, it is customary to administer the chemical during the entire period of organogenesis when the embryo is most susceptible. This period varies from one species to another. Such periods for some species of animals and related information are included in Table 11-1.

Observations

The Pregnant Animals   The animals should be examined daily for gross signs of toxicity, and any female that shows signs of impending abortion or premature delivery (e.g., vaginal bleeding) should be sacrificed and examined.

The Fetuses   Fetuses are usually surgically removed from the mother about one day prior to the expected delivery. This procedure is intended to avoid cannibalism and permit counting of resorption sites and dead fetuses.

The following observations are to be made and recorded:

Number of corpora lutea
Number and position of implantations
Number and position of resorptions

Table 11-1   Teratogenesis Studies on Various Animals

	Rat	Mouse	Hamster	Rabbit
Age of dam at start	100–120 d.	60–90 d.	60–90 d.	Adult virgin
Period of dosing[*]	d. 6–15	d. 6–15	d. 5–10	d. 6–18
Cesarean section[*]	d. 20	d. 17	d. 14	d. 29
Positive control[†]	ASA, 250 mg/kg	ASA, 150 mg/kg	ASA, 250 mg/kg	6-aminonicotinamide, 2.5 mg/kg

[*]D. 0 is when sperm is found in the vagina or, in the rabbit, the day of copulation or artificial insemination.

[†]ASA, acetylsalicyclic acid, which is a potent teratogen in certain laboratory animals, although only capable of inducing bleeding in human fetuses and only after large doses.

Number and position of dead fetuses
Number and position of live fetuses
Sex of each live fetus
Weight of each live fetus
Length (crown–rump) of each live fetus
Abnormalities of each fetus

Detailed Examinations These are required to determine the different types of abnormalities. Each fetus is examined for external defects. In addition, about two-thirds of random sampled fetuses are examined for skeletal abnormalities after staining with Alizarin red (Dawson, 1926). The remaining one-third of the fetuses are examined for visceral defects after fixation in Bouin's fluid and sectioned with razor blade (Wilson, 1965). With larger animals, e.g., dogs, pigs, and nonhuman primates, the skeletal structure is generally examined with X-ray instead of staining.

Delayed Effects With toxicants that are suspected of having effects on the fetal central nervous system or genitourinary system, a sufficient number of pregnant females are allowed to deliver their pups. These pups are nursed either by their biologic mothers, thus possibly being exposed to the toxicants via the milk, or by *foster mothers*. In the latter case, the potential effects of postnatal exposure are eliminated.

Neuromotor and behavioral tests may be used to detect CNS effects. These include posture, motor activity, coordination, endurance, vision, hearing, learning ability, response to foreign environment, mating behavior, and maternal behavior.

EVALUATION OF TERATOGENIC EFFECTS

Categories and Relative Significance

Aberrations As noted above, morphologic defects may involve external and/or internal structures. In addition, there may be functional abnormalities. Not all types of aberrations have the same significance. For example, supernumerary ribs and decreased, or abnormal, sternal ossification might have little or no visible effect on external morphology, functional activity, or survival of the fetus. These have been considered as *deviations*.

Malformations of doubtful significance include curly tail, straight legs, malrotated limbs and paws, wristdrop, protruding tongue, enlarged atria and/or ventricles, abnormal renal pelvic development, and translucent skin. In general, these have been characterized as *minor anomalies*. There are, at the other extreme, *major malformations* that are incompatible with survival, growth, development, fertility, and longevity, e.g., spina bifida, hydrocephalus.

In practice, the distinction between these categories is not always clear cut. It is then necessary to take other factors into consideration.

Resorption This is a manifestation of death of the conceptus. Although the site of resorption can be readily identified with a close examination of the uterus, the number of resorptions is more reliably determined by subtracting the total near-term offspring from the total implantations, as indicated by the number of corpora lutea. If there is an appreciable increase in the number of resorptions in the treated group, it may be necessary to alter the testing procedure to differentiate embryotoxicity from teratogenicity, e.g., by lowering the dose used to reduce the toxicity or shorten the exposure period of the dams.

Fetal Toxicity This may manifest as reduced body weight on nonviable fetus. This type of data is often useful as corroborating evidence in assessing the teratogenicity of the toxicant in question. With rabbits, the viability of fetus, if in question, may be determined by incubating it for 24 hours. With rodents, it may be advisable to repeat the test but allow the dams to deliver the pups.

Sources of Error

1 The animals used may exhibit an excessive number of spontaneous malformations or may be resistant to teratogenic effects. These errors can usually be assessed by the response of the animals to the negative and positive control agents.

2 Poor animal husbandry and mishandling of the animals may also result in an increased incidence of malformations.

3 The food consumption of the dams can be affected by the toxicant. This fact may then alter the body weight of the mothers and indirectly affect the fetuses.

4 Excessively large doses can result in many resorptions but few or no malformations. On the other hand, if the doses are too small, there may not be any evidence of teratogenicity.

5 Some teratogenic effects may be overlooked if only a cursory examination is carried out.

Analysis of the Results

In comparing the treated and control groups, the proper experimental unit is the litter rather than the individual fetuses, since each dam is an experimental unit (Weil, 1970). In other words, the numbers of litters with malformed fetuses, resorptions, or dead fetuses are the parameters to be used in statistical analysis. However, an increase in the average number of fetuses with defects per litter may provide corroborative evidence of teratogenicity.

If the results indicate a relationship between the doses and the response (incidence of malformation), it is generally justifiable to conclude that the agent is teratogenic under the specific experimental conditions.

When the incidence of malformation does not provide a definite conclusion, an analysis of the data from the historical controls may be valuable. Furthermore, a close examination of the data on the other parameters on the fetus and on the dam is sometimes useful.

Extrapolation to Humans

The results obtained in teratogenesis studies in animals cannot be readily extrapolated to humans. The lack of a suitable animal model is evidenced by the fact that the most potent human teratogen, thalidomide, which is effective at a dose of 0.5–1.0 mg/kg, has no teratogenic effects in rats and mice at 4000 mg/kg. Only moderate embryopathy is noted in rabbits. On the other hand, acetylsalicylic acid has a long history of safe use in human pregnancy but is a potent teratogen in rats, mice, and hamsters.

As pointed out by, among others, Harbison (1980), chemical teratogenesis is a challenging new area of toxicology. The mechanisms of teratogenesis and the differences in response among various species of animals are poorly understood. The causes of spontaneous congenital malformations in humans are unknown. More basic animal studies and prospective epidemiologic studies are required. At the same time, the astute clinician plays an important role in launching the first warning.

Nevertheless, since all chemicals that are teratogenic in humans have been shown to be active in certain animal models, it is prudent to carry out appropriate animal tests on all chemicals to which females of child-bearing age may be exposed. If positive results are obtained with a substance, especially when this is so in more than one species of animal, exposure of females of child-bearing age to this substance should be avoided, if possible. In assessing the teratogenic effects of a chemical, not only the incidence but also the severity of the aberrations should be taken into account (Khera, 1981).

IN VITRO TESTS

While these tests are not in routine use as yet, they show promise either as screening procedures, in pinpointing target organ, or in elaborating the mode of action of teratogens. Some of these tests are briefly described below; some details and references are provided by Saxén (1981).

Cell Culture

Cell cultures may be grown in suspension, as monolayer, or in various supporting materials. Teratogenic effects can be determined by a variety of endpoints. Because of the simplicity of the procedure, it can be used as a prescreen.

One type of endpoint involves analysis of the protein synthesized by the cultured cells, such as those from chick embryo. To ensure that the influence of bioactivation and placental barrier are taken into account, the cell culture is exposed to the chemical and its metabolites extracted from the amniotic fluid of pregnant mice that had been given the chemical.

Certain tumor cells in culture attach rapidly to a specially coated surface. It was found that chemicals shown to be teratogenic in animals generally inhibit the attachment of these cells. Another endpoint is alteration of cell differentiation by teratogenic chemicals. The alteration may be determined biochemically and morphologically.

Organ Culture

Metanephric kidney, developing tooth, and a number of other organs have been used for this purpose. The metanephric model is derived from 11-day mouse embryo metanephrenic mesenchyme and grown on a porous filter. An embryonic spinal cord is fixed on the opposite side of the filter as the inductor. It is removed after 24 hours, when the induction has taken place. The tissue then differentiates into glomeruli, proximal tubules, and distal tubules. A number of chemicals have been shown to reduce the number of tubules developed.

Organ cultures are too complex for use as a prescreen but appear useful for the study of the mode of action and target site of suspect chemicals.

Hydra Culture

Johnson and Gabel (1982) described a procedure using cultures of *Hydra attenuata* raised in laboratory conditions. Exposure of the adult hydra and artificial *embryos* (composed of randomly reaggregated cells of dissociated hydra) to chemicals causes various morphologic changes and death. The ratio of the lethal concentration in the embryo to that in the adult has been determined for several chemicals. These ratios show a good correlation with the ratios of the teratologic doses and the toxic doses in adult rodents. The procedure, therefore, also appears promising as a prescreen.

A much more extensive discussion of tests involving cultures of specific organs, tissues, whole embryos, and a variety of invertebrates are provided by WHO (1984).

APPENDIX 11-1: TERATOGENS IN ANIMAL MODELS

1 Physical agents: hypothermia and hyperthermia, hypoxia, radiation
2 Agents producing hypoxia: carbon monoxide, carbon dioxide
3 Infections: rubella viruses, syphilis
4 Dietary deficiency or excess: vitamins A, D, and E, ascorbic acid, nicotinamide, trace metals (Zn, Mn, Mg, Co)

5 Vitamin antagonists: antifolic drugs, 6-aminonicotinamide
6 Hormone deficiency or excess: cortisone, hydrocortisone, thyroxine, vasopressin, insulin, androgens, estrogens
7 Natural toxins: aflatoxin B_1, ochratoxin A, ergotamine, nicotine
8 Heavy metals: methyl mercury, phenylmercuric acetate, lead, thallium, strontium, selenium
9 Solvents: benzene, carbon tetrachloride, 1,1-dichloroethane, dimethyl sulfoxide, propylene glycol, xylene
10 Insecticides, herbicides, fungicides
11 Azo dyes: trypan blue, Evans blue, Niagara blue
12 Antibiotics: dactinomycin, penicillin, streptomycin, tetracyclines
13 Sulfonamides: sulfanilamide, hypoglycemic sulfonamides
14 Drugs and chemicals: caffeine, carbutamide, chlorcyclizine, chlorpromazine and derivatives, diphenylhydantoin, hydroxyurea, imipramine, meclizine, nitrosamines, pilocarpine, quinine, rauwolfia, thalidomide, triparanol, veratrum alkaloids, vinca alkaloids

REFERENCES

Collins, T. F. X., and Collins, E. V. (1976) Current methodology in teratology research. In: *New Concepts in Safety Evaluation, Part 1*. Eds. M. A. Mehlman, R. E. Shapiro, and H. Blumenthal. Washington, D.C.: Hemisphere.
Dawson, A. B. (1926) A note on the staining of the skeleton of cleared specimens with Alizarin Red S. *Stain Technol.* 1:123–124.
EPA (1982) *Health Effects Test Guidelines*. Washington, D.C.: Environmental Protection Agency.
Gregg, N. M. (1941) Congenital cataract following German measles in the mother. *Trans. Ophthalmol. Soc. Aust.* 3:35–46.
Hale, F. (1933) Pigs born without eyeballs. *J. Hered.* 24:105–106.
Harbison, R. D. (1980) Teratogens. In: *Casarett and Doull's Toxicology*. Eds. J. Doull, C. D. Klaassen, and M. O. Amdur. New York: Macmillan.
Health and Welfare, Canada (1973) *Carcinogenicity, Mutagenicity and Teratogenicity*. Ottawa: Department of Health and Welfare, Canada.
Johnson, E. M., and Gabel, B. E. G. (1982) Application of the hydra assay for rapid detection of developmental hazards. *J. Am. Coll. Toxicol.* 1(3):57–71.
Khera, K. S. (1981) Common fetal aberrations and their teratologic significance: A review. *Fundam. Appl. Toxicol.* 1:13–18.
Lenz, W. (1964) Chemicals and malformation in man, and congenital malformations. Papers and discussions presented at the Second International Medical Conference, New York, N.Y.
Lenz, W., and Knapp, K. (1962) Thalidomide embryopathy. *Arch. Environ. Health* 5:100–105.
Murphy, D. P. (1928) Ovarian irradiation—Its effect on the health of subsequent children: Review of the literature, experimental and clinical, with a report of 320 human pregnancies. *Surg. Gynecol. Obstet.* 47:201–215.

Saxén, L. (1981) Tests in vitro for teratogenicity. In: *Tests for Toxicity*. Ed. J. W. Gorrod. London: Taylor & Francis.

Shepard, T. H. (1980) *Catalog of Teratogenic Agents*, 3d ed. Baltimore: Johns Hopkins Univ. Press.

Timbrell, J. A. (1982) *Principles of Biochemical Toxicology*. London: Taylor & Francis.

Tuchmann-Duplessis, H. (1965) Design and interpretation of teratogenic tests. In: *Embryopathic Activity of Drugs*. Eds. J. M. Robson, F. M. Sullivan, and R. L. Smith. Boston: Little, Brown.

Warkany, J., and Shraffenberger, E. (1944) Congenital malformations induced in rats by maternal nutritional deficiency. VI. Preventive factor. *J. Nutr.* 27: 477–484.

Weil, C. (1970) Selection of the valid number of sampling units and a consideration of their combination in toxicological studies involving reproduction, teratogenesis or carcinogenesis. *Food Cosmet. Toxicol.* 8:177–182.

Wilson, J. G. (1965) Methods for administering agents and detecting malformations in experimental animal. In: *Teratology: Principles and Techniques*. Eds. J. G. Wilson and J. Warkany. Chicago: Univ. Chicago Press.

WHO (1967) *Principles for the Testing of Drugs for Teratogenicity*. WHO Tech. Rep. Ser. No. 365. Geneva: World Health Organization.

WHO (1984) *Principles for Evaluating Health Risks to Progeny Associated with Exposure to Chemicals During Pregnancy*. Environ. Health Criteria 30. Geneva: World Health Organization.

Part Three
Target Organs

Chapter 12

Respiratory System: Inhalation Toxicology

GENERAL CONSIDERATIONS

With industrialization, the respiratory system of humans is increasingly exposed to airborne toxicants. To study their health effects, a number of testing procedures have been devised, which are briefly described in this chapter.

It is important to note that the respiratory tract is a complex system. Furthermore, airborne substances exist in the form of gases, vapors, and liquid droplets and solid particulate matter of different sizes. The uptake and effects of inhaled toxicants therefore depend not only on their toxicologic nature but also on their physical characteristics.

The respiratory tract consists of the nasopharnx, the tracheal and bronchial tract, and the pulmonary acini, which are composed of respiratory bronchioles, alveolar ducts, and alveoli. The nasopharynx serves to remove large particles from the inhaled air, add moisture, and moderate the temperature. The tracheal and bronchial tract serves as the conducting airway to the alveoli. The trachea and bronchi are lined with ciliated epithelium and covered with a thin layer of mucus secreted by certain cells in the epithelial lining. This lining, with the cilia and mucus, can move particles deposited on the surface up to the mouth. The particle-containing mucus can then be eliminated from the respiratory tract by spitting or swallowing. However, minute liquid droplets and solid particulate matter can also be absorbed by diffusion and phagocytosis, as described in Chapter 2.

The pulmonary acini are the sites where oxygen and carbon dioxide are exchanged between the blood and the air and are the main sites of absorption of toxicants that exist in the form of gases and vapors. The alveoli are lined with epithelial cells, especially those of type I. These cells have a very thin cytoplasm (0.1–0.2 μm), but each covers a relatively large surface (2290 μm^2). The cuboidal (63 μm^2) type II cells can undergo mitosis and, in time, mature to type I cells. In addition, there are endothelial cells, macrophages, and fibroblasts (Menzel and McClellan, 1980).

Apart from its vital function in the exchange of oxygen and carbon dioxide, the respiratory system also regulates the blood concentrations of angiotensin, biogenic amines, and prostaglandins. Furthermore, it can excrete toxicants that have been absorbed from the lungs or via other routes, and it can, with its cyto-chrome P-450 system, biotransform many toxicants, some of which, such as paraquat, can yield reactive intermediates that are capable of binding to macro-molecules in the lungs.

CATEGORIES OF TOXIC EFFECTS

A toxicant may exert systemic effects after its absorption from the respiratory tract and distribution to other tissues, or it may induce local effects on the respiratory tract, or both. A toxicant may also affect the respiratory tract after exposure from other routes.

Systemic Effects

Many chemicals can be absorbed from the inspired air. After absorption, they are carried by the circulating blood to various parts of the body and exert their effects, such as general anesthesia.

Toxic gases can be absorbed from various parts of respiratory tract including the nasopharynx. The main site of absorption, however, is the alveoli, and the principle mechanism of absorption is simple diffusion. In addition, liquid aero-sols and solid particulate matter can also be absorbed via different mechanisms. Further details regarding the uptake of toxicants are given in Chapter 2.

Figure 12-1 shows the calculated average deposition curves for aerosols of various mass median aerodynamic diameters at different parts of the respiratory tract. These are the entire respiratory tract, nasopharynx, tracheobronchial tract, and pulmonary acini.

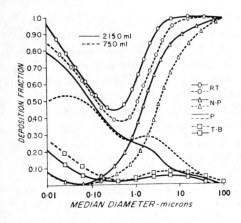

Figure 12-1 Calculated average deposition curves for aerosols for various mass median aerodynamic diameters at two different tidal volumes, i.e., 750 ml and 2150 ml. The respiratory rate is 15/min. (From Task Group on Lung Dynamics, 1966. Reproduced with permission of *Health Physics*, University of Florida.)

Effects on Lungs

A variety of pulmonary effects have been observed. These are briefly described under five categories. Additional details and references have been provided by Menzel and McClellan (1980).

Local Irritation   Ammonia and chlorine are classic examples of irritant gases. They cause bronchial constriction and edema, which result in dyspnea, but chronic effects are rare. Asenicals induce irritation on acute exposure; after prolonged exposure they can cause formation of lung cancer.

Cellular Damage and Edema   Toxic gases, such as ozone and nitrogen dioxide, can directly cause cellular damage, perhaps through peroxidation of cellular membranes. Edema ensues as a result of the increased permeability through the damaged membrane. The edematous fluid, however, accumulates in the airway instead of in the interstitial space, as is the case with other tissues. Such effects are also observed after inhalation of toxicants that exist in small particles, such as nickel carbonyl and certain beryllium and boron compounds.

Certain organic solvents, such as perchloroethylene and xylene, are rapidly absorbed after inhalation and distributed to various parts of the body including the liver, which is the major site of biotransformation. Part of the solvents reenters the lung through circulation and may form reactive metabolites, leading to covalent binding with macromolecules there. This process in turn produces cellular damage and edema.

Ipomeanol is a toxin produced by the mold *Fusarium solani*, grown on sweet potatoes. This toxin is interesting in that it causes necrosis of one type of cell only, namely the Clara cells. These cells are located at the boundary where alveolar ducts branch from bronchioles. They bioactivate the toxin to a reactive metabolite that binds to the macromolecules and causes cellular necrosis followed by edema. Death may ensue (Timbrell, 1982).

Fibrosis and Emphysema Pulmonary fibrosis is a serious, debilitating disease. Silicosis, with a history that goes back for thousands of years, is caused by crystalline forms of silica (silicon dioxide). Of the crystalline forms, quartz is the most stable. On heating, such as in volcanic eruption and mining, quartz may become tridymite or cristobolite. Both of these forms are more fibrogenic than quartz. The toxic effect stems from the rupture of the lysosomal membrane in a macrophage. The released lysosomal enzymes digest the macrophage, and this process, in turn, releases the silica from the lysed macrophage. And thus the process is repeated. It has been suggested that the damaged macrophage releases factors that stimulate the fibroblasts and the formation of collagen (Brian, 1980).

Another major cause of pulmonary fibrosis is asbestos. Asbestos refers to a large number of fibrous hydrated silicates of magnesium, calcium, and others. In addition, some of these mineral fibers, such as the blue asbestos (crocidolites), can cause bronchogenic carcinoma and mesothelioma. The white variety (chrysotile) appears to have no effect on the incidence of mesothelioma. The potency of asbestos seems related to the chemical and physical properties. Fibers of 5 μm in length and 0.3 μm in diameter appear to be most potent.

Other fibrogenic substances include coal dust, kaolin, talc, aluminum, beryllium, and carbides of tungsten, titanium, and tantalum.

Emphysema is also a debilitating disease. It may be induced by cigarette smoking or exposure to aluminum, cadmium oxide, or oxides of nitrogen, ozone, and others. It has been suggested that the elastic fibers surrounding and supporting the alveoli and bronchi may be damaged by the elastase released from polymorphonuclear granulocytes under certain conditions (Spitznagel et al., 1980).

Allergic Response This type of response is usually induced by spores of molds, bacterial contaminants, cotton dust, and so forth. A common chemical used in plastic industry, toluene diisocyanate (TDI), also produces hypersensitivity reaction. It is probable that this reactive chemical binds with proteins in the blood or lungs to form an antigen, which stimulates antibody formation. The major response is bronchoconstriction triggered by the reaction between the antigens and circulating or fixed antibodies. Long-term exposure may result in other pulmonary effects such as chronic bronchitis and fibrosis.

Lung Cancer Cigarette smoke contains a number of carcinogens and irritants. It is well established that cigarette smoking is the leading cause of lung cancer in many countries and that it increases the incidence of lung cancers among asbestos workers. Other causes of lung cancer include arsenic, chromates, nickel, uranium, coke oven emissions, and, as noted above, asbestos.

The effects of a number of occupationally inhaled toxicants, as adapted from Menzel and McClellan (1980), are listed in Appendix 12-1.

Effects on Upper Respiratory Tract

Large airborne particles in the inhaled air are mainly deposited in the nasal passages. They may cause hyperemia, squamous or transitional cell metaplasia, hyperplasia, ulceration, and, in certain cases, carcinoma. For example, nickel subsulfide, nickel oxide, and nickel usually exist in large particles during their production and mining; therefore, their effects are mainly on the nasal passage (NAS, 1975). The larynx is also a site of chemical carcinogenesis, e.g., asbestos and chromium. Inhalation of such vapors as sulfur dioxide and toluene may cause irritation of trachea and bronchi. Other toxic effects include deciliation, goblet cell hyperplasia, and squamous metaplasia (Cobb, 1981).

Effects after Other Routes of Exposure

The herbicide paraquat causes lung damages not only after exposure by inhalation but also after ingestion (Clark et al., 1966). Its storage in the lungs and its inherent toxicity are apparently the reasons for its pulmonary effects after noninhalation routes. In contrast, a closely related herbicide, diquat, although also toxic to cultured lung cells, is not toxic to the lungs either after inhalation or after ingestion. It is interesting that diquat is not retained by the lungs (Menzel and McClellan, 1980).

A number of drugs are known to induce pulmonary fibrosis in humans. These include bleomycin, busulfan, cyclophosphamide, gold salts, melphalan, methotrexate, and mitomycin. In these cases, there is an increase in interstitial collagen and in the number of type II epithelial cells. Methotrexate and streptomycin have been reported to cause pulmonary eosinophilia and phenylbutazone and oxyphenylbutazone to cause pulmonary edema (Cobb, 1981).

TESTING PROCEDURES

The local and systemic effects of toxicants resulting from their exposure via the respiratory tract is usually studied by mixing or suspending the toxicants in the air to be inhaled by the test subject. In exceptional cases the material on test is deposited, in liquid or solid form, in the respiratory tract.

Exposure Facilities

The systemic and local effects of toxicants administered to animals through the respiratory tract generally require elaborate facilities. The test animal may be placed in whole-body exposure chambers or exposed through the head or the nose only. Other systems have been designed to study the effects of toxicants through lung-only or partial lung exposure. The advantages and disadvantages of these approaches, as listed by Phalen (1976) are reproduced in Appendix

12-2. His article also provides references to detailed description of the procedures and facilities.

Whole-Body System Such a system typically consists of a chamber wherein the test animal is kept. The chamber is equipped with windows for observation of the test animal, and is connected to an air inlet and an air outlet. The toxicant, in the form of vapor or aerosol, is mixed with clean air and introduced into the chamber through the inlet. The outlet is usually connected to a filtering system to remove the toxicant from the exhaust before being released to the atmosphere. Typical systems have been described by Drew and Laskin (1973) and Phalen (1976). More recently, the design, operation, and characterization of a large, chronic inhalation exposure facility, with four 12.6 m³ exposure chambers, have been described (Schreck et al., 1981). Equipment for generating and controlling atmospheres in inhalation chambers has been described and compared by Rampy (1981).

MacFarland (1976) pointed out that the chamber should be at least 20 times the body volume of the test animal(s) that is to be kept in the chamber. Smaller chambers tend to cause significant reduction of the concentration of the toxicant and may increase the temperature inside. He also emphasized the need to ensure satisfactorily uniform distribution of the airborne substance in designing the shape of the chamber and that the wall of the chamber should be made of materials (such as stainless steel and glass) that absorb only a minimal amount of the toxicant and can be readily cleaned.

Head- and Nose-Exposure Systems These systems have the advantages of (1) avoiding absorption of the toxicant deposited on the fur, either directly through the skin or indirectly through the gastrointestinal tract when the animal grooms itself and (2) requiring a more limited quantity of the test material. However, the animals must be restrained. Moreover, fitting the head or nostrils of the animals to the apparatus requires some skill and time. A number of such systems have been developed and the references to their descriptions are also given in a WHO document (1978). Many of these systems have been used to study the effects of cigarette smoke in various species of animals, including donkeys. A recent article describes a method for chronic nose-only exposure of laboratory animals to inhaled fibrous aerosols (Smith et al., 1981).

Choice of Animals

The commonly used experimental animals are rats, dogs, and monkeys. Others include mice, hamsters, guinea pigs, rabbits, miniature pigs, and donkeys. The choice should be based on a number of criteria, such as the anatomic similarity of the respiratory tract of humans and that of the animal. Appendix 12-3 provides the comparative anatomy of the lung of a number of animals and of humans. It may be noted that monkeys are distinctly different from humans in spite of their phylogenetic proximity. Horses, presumably donkeys also, are very similar to humans in this respect. Other factors, which may be more important, are the similarity of their biochemical and physiologic responses to those of humans and an abundance of experimental results, which permits comparison between the toxicities of various chemicals.

It has been well documented in epidemiologic studies that people with preexisting cardiopulmonary diseases are at special risk during air pollution episodes. To simulate this condition, papain-induced emphysematous animals have been used (Gross et al., 1965).

Doses

Definition of Dose In general, the dose is the amount of a substance that is administered to an organism. The amount is readily ascertained when the substance is given by a route such as oral, subcutaneous, intravenous, or intraperitoneal. This definition is not applicable to exposure by inhalation, because the amount that is retained in the animal depends on the concentration of the toxicant in the inhaled air as well as the duration of the exposure. In other words, the dose might be *expressed* as the product of the concentration (C) and the time (t). It has been recognized that for a fixed C × t product the response will be the same. However, this rule is not valid when either C or t is an extreme value. For example, if C is too small, generally no response will be elicited no matter how long the animal is exposed to it.

Procedures have been suggested for measuring the retained dose (Leong and MacFarland, 1965). However, there are great variations between animals, especially rodents. Part of the reason lies in their different abilities to avoid the uptake of obnoxious materials (Alarie, 1966).

In most inhalation studies the retained doses are not estimated. Instead, the duration of exposure is kept constant whereas the test animals are exposed to different concentrations of a toxicant. For example, in acute median lethality studies, the animals are exposed, as a rule for 4 hours. In longer-term studies either a *continuous* (23 hours/day) or an *intermittent* (8 hours/day, 5 days/week) exposure scheme is adopted, the former being designed to simulate the exposure to environmental pollutants and the latter, industrial situations.

Selection of Doses In acute lethality studies, one concentration should be aimed at causing the death of about 50% of the animals. At least two other concentrations are selected, one killing more than 50% but less than 90%, and the other killing 10–50% of the animals.

In longer-term studies, at least three concentrations should be selected. The highest concentration is intended to cause some toxic effects and the lowest concentrations should have no observable effects.

Maintenance of Preselected Concentrations The nominal concentration is determined by dividing the amount of the agent used in the system that generates the airborne toxicant by the air flow through the exposure chamber. The actual concentrations, however, is often not the same as the nominal concentration. The former is determined by actual analysis of samples of the chamber air taken near the breathing zone of the animals. Since the actual concentrations usually vary through an exposure period, it is necessary to analyze a number of samples taken at appropriate time intervals. The exposure facility should be so designed as to minimize the range of variations. A number of references on exposure systems, generating systems, and sampling methods are provided by WHO (1978).

Duration of Exposure

For acute LC_{50} determinations (LC_{50} is the concentration that will cause the death of 50% of the animals at a specific duration of exposure), the duration of exposure is usually between 1 and 4 hours. In short-term studies the duration is usually 30 or 90 days, and in long-term studies it is 1 year or more. The repeated exposures are either on a continuous or intermittent basis, as discussed above.

The duration of each exposure is generally considered as between the time the toxicant is introduced into the chamber to the time the generator is turned off. However, the animal is kept in the chamber while the clean air inflow is continued. As shown in Fig. 12-2, the exposure starts at time t_a and stops at t_c.

The duration between t_a and t_{99} depends on the ratio of the volume of the chamber to the flow of air through the chamber. If the ratio is 1, t_{99} is 4.6 minutes. If the ratio is 5, t_{99} is $5 \times 4.6 = 23$ minutes.

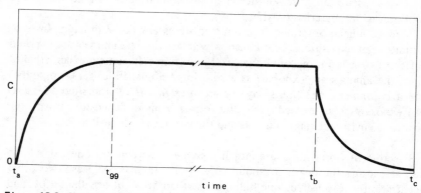

Figure 12-2 The buildup and decay of a pollutant in a chamber. Exposure starts at t_a and stops at t_c, but the flow of the toxicant is terminated at t_b. The duration of exposure is recorded as from t_a to t_b; the extra exposure from t_b to t_c is intended to compensate for the exponential buildup of the toxicant in the chamber from t_a to t_{99}. (From MacFarland, 1976.)

Observations and Examinations

✓ **General** These include body weight and food consumption, general observations, laboratory tests, and postmortem examinations. Some details on these are given in Chapter 8.

Respiratory Functions Tests on these functions are often carried out because of their greater sensitivity than morphologic changes and because of their ability to detect reversible effects. As a result, (these tests might be used in studies in humans, thereby allowing a more valid comparison between humans and the experimental animals with respect to their relative susceptibility to the toxic effects of the substance being tested.)

Respiratory frequency is a sensitive indicator of local irritation and is often concentration-related. Certain gases, e.g., ozone and nitrogen dioxide, increase the frequency, whereas others, e.g., sulfur dioxide and formaldehyde, decrease it.

Mechanics of respiration can be measured in terms of pulmonary flow resistance and pulmonary compliance. An increase in pulmonary flow resistance can result from bronchoconstriction, swelling of the respiratory mucosa, or an increase in mucous secretion. Pulmonary compliance is decreased by fibrosis, and it is increased in emphysema because of loss of supportive connective tissue. References to their measurements are given in a WHO document (1978).

Respiratory efficiency can be estimated by measuring oxygen and carbon dioxide in the blood or by measuring the rate at which inhaled carbon monoxide is taken into the blood (Cobb, 1981).

Morphologic and Biochemical Changes As described above, various morphologic changes can result from inhalation exposure to toxicants. These include local irritation, cellular damage, edema, fibrosis, and neoplasms. In addition, toxicants can cause a number of other types of morphologic changes such as inflammation, hyperplasia, and emphysema, as shown in Appendix 12-1.

Some examinations are especially useful. For example, lung-weight increases are indicators of vascular congestion, edema, or increase in connective tissue. Washings of the lung can provide information on the cell number, type, and morphology as well as on noncellular components, especially the enzyme content. Furthermore, the collagen content can be estimated by determining hydroxyproline or prolylhydroxylase (Cobb, 1981).

EVALUATION

Analyses of the data relating to the effects and the dose are essentially the same as those following other routes of administration, with the exception that the dose is generally handled differently.

As noted above, while the retained dose after exposure by inhalation can be estimated, the common practice is to use the concentration instead. Thus, the results of acute median lethality studies are expressed as LC_{50}. The LC_{50} values of various compounds can be compared, provided the same duration of exposure was used in the inhalation studies.

The determination of the dose-effect and the dose-response relationships can also be done in the conventional manner, using concentrations instead of doses. The procedure employed in the estimation of the *no-effect level*, as described in Chapter 7, can also be adopted in inhalation studies.

Whereas the concentration can be readily expressed with gases and vapors, the *effective* concentration of aerosols is influenced by the particle size, which can greatly influence the penetration and absorption of the material. Thus, when reporting inhalation studies, it is necessary to provide information on the median particle size and their geometric standard deviations (Chapter 2 and Fig. 12-2).

IN VITRO TESTS

In order to conduct more definitive studies on the effects of toxicants on the respiratory system, various in vitro systems have been developed.

Isolated Perfused Lung

Lungs isolated from rabbits or rats are perfused with heparinized blood at a constant pressure and ventilated with positive pressure through the trachea or negative pressure from outside of the lung. A constant blood flow can be maintained over a period of several hours. The system is especially useful in determining nonrespiratory functions of the lung. For example, the levels of the endogenous hormones and vasoactive amines can be readily determined in the exudate. Furthermore, the pulmonary metabolism of a toxicant can be ascertained by adding it to the perfusate and analyzing the exudate for the toxicant and its metabolite. Some details and references are provided by Anderson and Eling (1976) and Roth (1980).

Tracheal Explants

The effects of toxic gases and vapors can be assessed on the trachea removed from animals, such as rats, that have been exposed to toxicants. When incubated in a tissue culture medium the trachea will continue to secrete mucous glycoproteins. The rate of secretion can be affected by exposure to toxicants. For example, tracheal explants taken from rats exposed to ozone at 0.8 ppm showed an increased rate of secretion, but those from rats exposed to 0.5 ppm ozone or 1.1 mg/m^3 sulfuric acid did not. Exposure to the combination, however, induced significantly greater rates of secretion (Last and Kaizer, 1980).

Isolated Cells

Various types of cells from the respiratory system have been isolated and cultured. These include the epithelial cells of the trachea and the lung tissue as well as the endothelial cells. Isolated cultured cells show promise of becoming useful tools in toxicology of the respiratory system. Reiser and Last (1979), for example, pointed out the importance of pulmonary alveolar macrophages and fibroblasts in the development of fibrosis in chronic silicosis. They also noted the likelihood of involvement of other cell types, the precise role of which awaits further studies with isolated cells.

APPENDIX 12-1: SITE OF ACTION AND PULMONARY DISEASE PRODUCED BY SELECTED OCCUPATIONALLY INHALED TOXICANTS

Toxicant	Common name of disease	Site of action	Acute effect	Chronic effect
Aluminum	Aluminosis	Upper airways, alveolar interstitium	Cough, shortness of breath	Interstitial fibrosis
Aluminum abrasives	Shaver's disease, corundum smelter's lung, bauxite lung	Alveoli	Alveolar edema	Fibrotic thickening of alveolar walls, interstitial fibrosis and emphysema
Ammonia		Upper airways	Immediate upper and lower respiratory tract irritation, edema	Chronic bronchitis
Arsenic		Upper airways	Bronchitis	Lung cancer, bronchitis, laryngitis
Asbestos	Asbestosis	Parenchyma		Pulmonary fibrosis, pleural calcification, lung cancer, pleural mesothelioma
Beryllium	Berylliosis	Alveoli	Severe pulmonary edema, pneumonia	Pulmonary fibrosis, progressive dyspnea, interstitial granulomatosis, cor pulmonale
Boron		Alveoli	Edema and hemorrhage	
Cadmium oxide		Alveoli	Cough, pneumonia	Emphysema, cor pulmonale
Carbides of tungsten, titanium, tantalum	Hard metal disease	Upper and lower airways	Hyperplasia and metaplasia of bronchial epithelium	Fibrosis, peribronchial and perivascular fibrosis

Source: Menzel and McClellan, 1980.

Appendix 12-1 (*Continued*)

Toxicant	Common name of disease	Site of action	Acute effect	Chronic effect
Chlorine		Upper airways	Cough, hemoptysis, dyspnea, tracheo-bronchitis, broncho-pneumonia	
Chromium (VI)		Nasopharynx, upper airways	Nasal irritation, bronchitis	Lung tumors and cancers
Coal dust	Pneumoconiosis	Lung parenchyma, lymph nodes, hilus		Pulmonary fibrosis
Coke oven emissions		Upper airways		Tracheobronchial cancers
Cotton dust	Byssinosis	Upper airways	Tightness in chest, wheezing, dyspnea	Reduced pulmonary function, chronic bronchitis
Hydrogen fluoride		Upper airways	Respiratory irritation, hemorrhagic pulmonary edema	
Iron oxides	Siderotic lung disease: Silver finisher's lung, hematite miner's lung, arc welders's lung	Silver finisher's: pulmonary vessels and alveolar walls; hematite miner's: upper lobes, bronchi and alveoli; arc welder's: bronchi	Cough	Silver finisher's: subpleural and perivascular aggregations of macrophages; hematite miner's: diffuse fibrosis-like pneumoconiosis; arc welder's: bronchitis
Kaolin	Kaolinosis	Lung parenchyma, lymph nodes, hilus		Pulmonary fibrosis
Manganese	Manganese pneumonia	Lower airways and alveoli	Acute pneumonia, often fatal	Recurrent pneumonia
Nickel		Parenchyma (NiCO), nasal mucosa (Ni_2S_3), bronchi (NiO)	Pulmonary edema, delayed by 2 days (NiCO)	Squamous cell carcinoma of nasal cavity and lung

Appendix 12-1 (*Continued*)

Toxicant	Common name of disease	Site of action	Acute effect	Chronic effect
Osmium tetraoxide		Upper airways	Bronchitis, broncho- pneumonia	
Oxides of nitrogen		Terminal respiratory bronchi and alveoli	Pulmonary congestion and edema	Emphysema
Ozone		Terminal respiratory bronchi and alveoli	Pulmonary edema	Emphysema
Phosgene		Alveoli	Edema	Bronchitis
Perchloro- ethylene			Pulmonary edema	
Silica	Silicosis, pneumoconiosis	Lung parenchyma, lymph nodes, hilus		Pulmonary fibrosis
Sulfur dioxide		Upper airways	Bronchoconstric- tion, cough, tightness in chest	
Talc	Talcosis	Lung parenchyma, lymph nodes		Pulmonary fibrosis
Tin	Stanosis	Bronchioles and pleura		Widespread mottling of X-ray without clinical signs
Toluene		Upper airways	Acute bronchitis, bronchospasm, pulmonary edema	
Vanadium		Upper and lower airways	Upper airway irritation and mucus production	Chronic bronchitis
Xylene		Lower airways	Pulmonary edema	

APPENDIX 12-2: Comparative Evaluation of Inhalation Exposure Methods and Some Design Considerations Associated with Each Method

Mode of exposure	Advantages	Disadvantages	Design considerations
Chambers (whole-body)	Variety and number of animals Chronic studies Minimum restraint Large data base Controllable environment Impressive	Messy Multiple routes of exposure: skin, eyes, oral (food, water) Variability of dose Can not pulse exposure easily Inefficient Poor contact between animals and investigators Expensive	Clean air Inert materials Losses Even distribution in space and time Sampling Animal care Observation Noise, vibration, humidity Air temperature Safe exhaust Loading Reliability
Head only	Good for repeated exposure Limited routes of entry into animal More efficient dose delivery	Stress to animal Losses can be large Seal around neck Labor in loading/unloading	Even distribution Pressure fluctuations Sampling and losses Air temperature, humidity Animal comfort Animal restraint
Nose/mouth only	Exposure limited to mouth and respiratory tract Uses less material (efficient) Containment of material Can pulse the exposure	Stress to animal Seal about face Effort to expose large number of animals	Pressure fluctuations Body temperature Sampling Seals Animal comfort Losses in plumbing/masks
Lung only	Precision of dose One route of exposure Uses less material (efficient) Can pulse the exposure	Technically difficult Anesthesia or tracheostomy Limited to small numbers Bypasses nose Artifacts in deposition and response Technically more difficult	Air humidity/temperature Stress to the animal Physiologic support
Partial lung	Precision of total dose Localization of dose Can achieve very high local doses Unexposed control tissue from same animal	Anesthesia Placement of dose Difficulty in interpretation of results Technically difficult Possible redistribution of material within lung	Stress to animal Physiologic support

Source: Phalen, 1976.

	Humans	Mouse, rat, gerbil, hamster, guinea pig, rabbit	Dog, cat	Ox, sheep pig	Macaque, monkey	Horse	Ferret
Pleuras	Thick	Thin (Refs. 5, 9)	Thin (Refs. 4, 9)	Thick (Refs. 4, 9)	Thin	Thick	
Interlobular connective tissue	Extensive, partially surrounds many lobules	Little, if any	Little, if any	Extensive surrounds many lobules completely	Little	Extensive, partially surrounds many lobules	
Bronchioles: Nonrespiratory, nonalveolarized	Several generations	Several generations	Fewer generations	Several generations	Fewer generations, commonly only one	Several generations	Several generations
	TB ends in respiratory bronchioles	TB ends in avelolar ducts or very short respiratory bronchioles	TB ends in respiratory bronchioles	TB ends in alveolar ducts or very short respiratory bronchioles	TB ends in respiratory bronchioles		TB ends in respiratory bronchioles
Respiratory	Several generations	Absent or a single short generation	Several generations; typical distal airway	Absent or single short generation	Several generations, typical distal airway	Not common	Several generations

Source: Tyler, 1983. (Reproduced with permission of the American Review of Respiratory Disease.)
TB = terminal bronchiole.

REFERENCES

Alarie, Y. (1966) Irritating properties of airborne materials to the upper respiratory tract. *Arch. Environ. Health* 13:433–449.

Anderson, M. W., and Eling, T. E. (1976) Studies on the uptake, metabolism, and release of endogenous and exogenous chemicals by the use of the isolated perfused lung. *Environ. Health Perspect.* 16:77–81.

Brian, J. D. (1980) Macrophage damage in relation to the pathogenesis of lung diseases. *Environ. Health Perspect.* 35:21–28.

Cobb, L. M. (1981) Pulmonary toxicity. In: *Testing for Toxicity*. Ed. J. Gorrod. London: Taylor & Francis.

Clark, D. G., McElligott, T. F., and Hurst, E. W. (1966) The toxicity of paraquat. *Br. J. Ind. Med.* 23:126–132.

Drew, R. T., and Laskin, S. (1973) Environmental inhalation chambers. In: *Methods of Animal Experimentation*. Ed. W. I. Day. New York: Academic Press.

Gross, P., Pfitzer, E. A., Tolker, E., Babyak, M. A., and Kaschak, M. (1965) Experimental emphysema: Its production with papain in normal and silicotic rats. *Arch. Environ. Health* 11:50–58.

Last, J. A., and Kaizer, T. (1980) Mucus glycoprotein secretion by tracheal explants: Effect of pollutants. *Environ. Health Perspect.* 35:131–137.

Leong, K. J., and MacFarland, H. N. (1965) Pulmonary dynamics and retention of toxic gases–I. Sulfur dioxide: Concentration and duration effects in rats. *Arch. Environ. Health 11:555–563.*

MacFarland, H. N. (1976) Respiratory toxicology. In: Essays in Toxicology, Vol. 7. Ed. W. J. Hayes, New York: Academic Press.

Menzel, D. B., and McClellan, R. O. (1980) Toxic responses of the respiratory system. In: *Casarett and Doull's Toxicology: The Basic Science of Poisons*, 2d ed. Eds. J. Doull, C. D. Klaassen, and M. O. Amdur. New York: Macmillan.

National Academy of Sciences (NAS) (1975) *Nickel.* Washington, D.C.: National Academy of Sciences.

Phalen, R. F. (1976) Inhalation exposure of animals. *Environ. Health Perspect.* 16:17–24.

Rampy, L. W. (1981) Generating and controlling atmospheres in inhalation chambers. In: *Scientific Considerations in Monitoring and Evaluating Toxicological Research*. Ed. E. J. Gralla. Washington, D.C.: Hemisphere.

Reiser, K. M., and Last, J. A. (1979) Silicosis and fibrogenesis: Fact and artifact. *Toxicology* 13:51–72.

Roth, J. A. (1980) Use of perfused lung in biochemical toxicology. *Rev. Biochem. Toxicol.* 1:287–309.

Schreck, R. M., Chan, T. L., and Soderholm, S. C. (1981) Design operation and characterization of large volume exposure chambers. In: *Proceedings of the Inhalation Toxicology and Technology Symposium*. Ed. B. K. J. Leong. Ann Arbor, Mich.: Ann Arbor Science.

Smith, D. M., Ortiz, L. W., Anchuleta, R. F., Spalding, J. F., Tillery, M. I., Ettinger, H. J., and Thomas, R. G. (1981) A method for chronic nose-exposures of laboratory animals to inhaled fibrous aerosols. In: *Proceedings of Inhalation Toxicology and Technology Symposium*. Ed. B. K. J. Leong. Ann Arbor, Mich.: Ann Arbor Science.

Spitznagel, J. K., Moderzakowski, M. C., Pryzwansky, K. B., and MacRae, E. K. (1980) Neutral proteasus of human polymorphonuclear granulocytes: Putative mediators of pulmonary damage. *Environ. Health Perspect.* 35: 29–38.

Task Group on Lung Dynamics (1966) *Health Phys.* 12:173.

Timbrell, J. A. (1982) *Principles of Biochemical Toxicology*. London: Taylor & Francis.

Tyler, W. S. (1983) Comparative lung biology. *Am. Rev. Respir. Dis.* 128:S34.

WHO (1978) Inhalation exposure. In: *Principles and Methods for Evaluating the Toxicity of Chemicals. Part I*. Environmental Health Criteria 6. Geneva: World Health Organization.

Chapter 13

Toxicology of the Liver

GENERAL CONSIDERATIONS

The liver is the largest and metabolically the most complex organ in the body. It is involved in the metabolism of nutrients as well as most drugs and toxicants. The latter type of substances can usually be detoxified, but many of them can be bioactivated and become more toxic.

Hepatocytes (hepatic parenchymal cells) comprise the bulk of the organ. They are responsible for the liver's central role in metabolism. These cells lie between the blood-filled sinusoids and the biliary passages. Kupffer cells line the hepatic sinusoids and constitute an important part of the reticuloendothelial system of the body. The blood is supplied through the portal vein and hepatic artery, and it is drained through the hepatic vein into the vena cava. The biliary passages begin as tiny bile canaliculi formed by adjacent parenchymal cells. The canaliculi coalesce into ductules, interlobular bile ducts, and larger hepatic ducts. The main hepatic duct joins the cystic duct from the gallbladder to form the common bile duct, which drains into the duodenum.

The toxicology of liver is complicated by the variety of liver injuries and by the different mechanisms through which the injuries are induced. The types of injury, the underlying mechanisms, and the morphologic and biochemical changes are described and discussed.

The liver is often the target organ for a number of reasons. Most toxicants enter the body via the gastrointestinal tract, and after absorption they are carried by the hepatic portal vein to the liver. The liver has a high concentration of binding sites. It also has a high concentration of xenobiotic-metabolizing enzymes, some of which activate the toxicants to induce lesions locally. The fact that hepatic lesions are often centrilobular has been attributed to the higher concentration of cytochrome P-450 there (Bridges, 1981). In addition, the relatively lower concentration of glutathione there, compared to that in other parts of the liver, may also play a role (Smith et al., 1979).

TYPES OF LIVER INJURY

Fatty Liver (Steatosis)

(A fatty liver is one that contains more than 5% lipid by weight) The presence of an excess stainable fat in such liver is demonstrable histochemically. The lesion can be acute, such as that induced by ethionine, phosphorus, or tetracycline. Ethanol and methotrexate can cause either acute or chronic lesions. Some toxicants, e.g., tetracycline, produce many small fat droplets in a cell, whereas others, e.g., ethanol, induce large fat droplets, which displace the nucleus.

Although lipid accumulation in the liver is the common endpoint of these toxicants, the underlying mechanisms are varied. (Accumulation of lipid in the liver can result from an oversupply of free fatty acids from adipose tissue.) Physical stress (e.g., noise), hypoxia, and chemical stress (e.g., DDT, nicotine) can stimulate the pituitary-adrenal axis and trigger massive release of catecholamine, which in turn mobilizes depot fat.)

Perhaps the most common mechanism is impairment of the release of hepatic triglyceride to the plasma. Since hepatic triglyceride is secreted only when it is combined with lipoprotein [forming *very low density lipoprotein* (VLDL)], accumulation of hepatic lipid can occur as a result of a number of mechanisms (Plaa, 1980):

1 Inhibition of the synthesis of the protein moiety of lipoprotein (e.g., carbon tetrachloride, ethionine)

2 Depressed conjugation of triglyceride with lipoprotein (e.g., carbon tetrachloride)

3 Loss of potassium from hepatocytes, resulting in an interference of transfer of the VLDL across the cell membrane (e.g., ethionine)

4 Impaired oxidation of lipids by mitochondria (e.g., ethanol)

5 Inhibition of the synthesis of phospholipids, a vital part of the VLDL (e.g., choline deficiency, orotic acid)

Liver Necrosis

Liver necrosis involves the death of hepatocytes. The necrosis can be focal (central, mid-zonal, peripheral) or massive. It is usually an acute injury. A number of chemicals have been demonstrated or reported to cause liver necrosis (Zimerman, 1982). It is a serious toxic manifestation but is not necessarily critical because of the remarkable regenerating capacity of the liver.

Cell death occurs along with rupture of the plasma membrane. No ultrastructural changes of the membrane per se have been detected prior to its rupture. There are, however, a number of changes that precede the cell death. Early morphologic changes include cytoplasmic edema, dilatation of endoplasmic reticulum, and disaggregation of polysomes. There is an accumulation of triglycerides as fat droplets in the cells. Late changes are progressive swelling of mitochondria with cristae disruption, cytoplasmic swelling, dissolution of organelles and nucleus, and rupture of plasma membrane (see Bridges et al., 1983).

The biochemical changes are complex, and various heptotoxicants apparently act through different mechanisms. Carbon tetrachloride (CCl_4) is the most extensively studied hepatotoxicant. It acts primarily through its reactive metabolite, the trichloromethyl radical (Recknagel and Glende, 1973), which covalently binds with proteins and unsaturated lipids and induces lipid peroxidation. Subcellular membranes are rich in such lipids and are therefore susceptible (see Fig. 2-1). These biochemical reactions are followed by a series of disturbances as shown in Fig. 13-1. The chemical alterations in the membrane may be the cause of its rupture.

Recknagel et al. (1982), however, suggested that microsomal lipid peroxidation might lead to a depression of microsomal Ca^{2+} pump resulting in an early

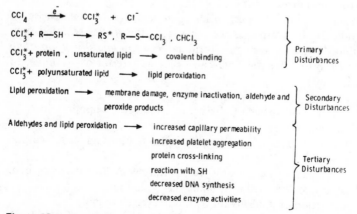

Figure 13-1 Sequence of cellular events following the biotransformation of carbon tetrachlorode to a reactive metabolite. (From Timbrell, 1982.)

disturbance of liver cell Ca^{2+} homeostasis, which might then induce cell death. In addition, Shah et al. (1979) suggested that the toxicity of CCl_4 might be mediated through another metabolite, i.e., phosgene.

Because of the complexity of the effects, Hewitt et al. (1982) studied the potentiation of the hepatotoxicity of CCl_4 by 1,3-butanediol. They suggested that the potentiation is mediated through a variety of routes, e.g., increasing the bioactivation of CCl_4, favoring the formation of phosgene over CCl_3^*, depleting hepatic glutathione and enhancing the susceptibility of subcellular organelles.

A number of chemically related compounds, e.g., chloroform, tetrachloro-ethane, and carbon tetrabromide, as well as phosphorus appear to act in similar ways. So do a number of other chemicals. However, at low doses, the reactive metabolite of acetaminophen conjugates with sulfate and glutathione. With increasing doses the level of glutathione reduces, and the covalent binding of the chemical to the proteins rises, as dramatically shown in Fig. 3-2. Bromobenzene is also bioactivated in the liver. Its 3,4-epoxide covalently binds to proteins and lipids and causes necrosis (see also Chapter 3). Other examples include isoniazid and iproniazid, both of which undergo bioactivation and form metabolites that bind with macromolecules and cause necrosis (Mitchell et al., 1976).

There are other chemicals, such as antimetabolites, that exert their toxicity through interference with metabolic pathways. Phalloidin acts via attachment to membrane receptors. Additional details and relevant references are provided by Zimmerman (1982).

While inhibition of protein synthesis is a significant effect in necrosis, this is not always true. For example, ethionine and cycloheximide inhibit protein synthesis, but this may not be followed by necrosis, and beryllium causes necrosis without early inhibition of protein synthesis. It is also interesting to note that while cycloheximide can cause liver necrosis, it may actually protect the liver from the toxic effect of CCl_4 (Farber, 1975). This phenomenon has been explained on the basis that CCl_4 only inhibits single units of ribosomes and has no effect on the polysomes induced by cycloheximide.

Other biochemical changes include depletion of adenosine triphosphate (ATP), loss of calcium ion, shifts of the Na^+ and K^+ balance between hepatocytes and blood, depletion of glutathione, damage to cytochrome P-450, and loss of NAD and NADP (Kulkarni and Hodgson, 1980; Timbrell, 1982).

Cholestasis

This type of liver damage, usually acute, is less common than fatty liver and necrosis, and it is more difficult to induce in animals. Certain bile salts, such as lithocholic acid and taurolithocholic acid, can interact with the canalicular membrane, thereby affecting the bile flow (Boyer et al., 1977). Taurolithocholate is poorly water soluble and its precipitation in the biliary tract can thus block the bile flow (Javitt and Emerson, 1968).

ANIT (α-naphthylisocyanate) can induce cholestasis and hyperbilirubinemia, as well as bromsulphthalein (BSP) retention and inhibition of microsomal mixed-function oxygenases. Reduction of biliary excretory activity appears to be the predominant mechanism for the cholestasis. Furthermore, ANIT seems to alter ductular cell permeability (Plaa and Priestly, 1976).

A number of anabolic and contraceptive steroids have been found to cause cholestasis and hyperbilirubinemia associated with canalicular bile plugs (Imai and Hayashi, 1970). Ethinyl estradiol and chlorpromazine seem to impair the permeability of the biliary tract, thus reducing bile salt-independent bile flow.

There are different mechanisms for cholestasis:

1. Impaired canalicular membrane function, e.g., ANIT, taurolithocholate
2. Intracanalicular precipitation, e.g., taurocholate, chlorpromazine, erythromycin lactobionate
3. Hypertrophic hypoactive smooth endoplasmic reticulum, e.g., bile salts, ANIT
4. Altered ductular cell permeability, e.g., ANIT
5. Impaired bile salt-independent canalicular bile flow, e.g., chlorpromazine, ethinyl estradiol (Plaa and Priestly, 1976).

Cirrhosis

Cirrhosis is characterized by the presence of septae of collagen distributed throughout most of the liver. Separated by these fibrous sheaths, clusters of hepatocytes appear as nodules.

The pathogenesis is not fully understood, but in a majority of cases, cirrhosis seems to originate from single-cell necrosis associated with a deficiency in the repair mechanism. This condition then leads to fibroblastic activity and scar formation. Inadequate blood flow in the liver may be a contributing factor.

Several chemical carcinogens and long-term administration of CCl_4 can induce cirrhosis in animals. The most important cause of human cirrhosis is chronic ingestion of alcoholic beverages. This pathologic condition can be induced in animals only with ethanol in combination with diets deficient in choline, proteins, methionine, vitamin B_{12}, and folic acid. Since this type of nutritional deficiency is common in alcoholism, Hartroft (1975) suggested the nutritional deficiency as the primary cause. Lieber and DiCarli (1976) were able to induce cirrhosis in baboons with ethanol alone and claimed, therefore, that alcohol has hepatotoxicity.

Viral-like Hepatitis

A clinical syndrome indistinguishable from viral hepatitis has been known to be associated with various drugs. In general, they have the following characteristics (Plaa, 1980; Zimmerman, 1982):

1. Such liver injuries are not demonstrable in animals.
2. The effects in humans do not seem to be related to the dose.
3. The latent period varies greatly.
4. The toxicity is manifest in only a few susceptible individuals.
5. The histologic picture is more variable.
6. The patients usually show other signs of hypersensitivity and sometimes respond to a challenge dose.
7. Fever, rash, and eosinophilia are present in many cases.

The clinical picture may vary from patient to patient. For example, among those with halothane-induced hepatotoxicity, 50% of the patients had signs of typical hypersensitivity reaction: fever, eosinophilia, prior exposure to this anesthetic. Others did not exhibit these signs and the livers of fatal cases showed lesions similar to those induced by CCl_4 (Zimmerman, 1982).

Carcinogenesis

Hepatocellular carcinoma and cholangiocarcinoma are the most common types of primary malignant neoplasms of the liver. Others include angiosarcoma, glandular carcinoma, trabecular carcinoma, and undifferentiated liver cell carcinoma. The significance of adenoma, focal basophilic hyperplasia, and hyperplastic nodule is as yet uncertain, whereas bile duct hyperplasia is likely to be a physiologic response to toxic exposure (Newberne, 1982).

As discussed in Chapter 9, a large number of toxicants are known to induce liver cancers in animals. However, their carcinogenicity in humans with respect to liver has not been well established (Wogan, 1976). On the other hand, the role of vinyl chloride in causing angiosarcoma in humans is beyond doubt.

HEPATOTOXICANTS

Some of the liver injuries described above, namely, steatosis, necrosis, cirrhosis, and neoplasia, have a number of common features. These injuries are relatively easily produced in experimental animals. Many toxicants can induce several types of such injuries. For example, steatosis, necrosis, and cirrhosis can result from exposure to CCl_4 (and related chemicals such as chloroform), aflatoxins, and phosphorus. Aflatoxins and dioxins can induce necrosis, cirrhosis, and neoplasm. Steatosis and cirrhosis are seen after exposure to ethanol, and bromobenzene is known to induce necrosis and cirrhosis.

Cholestasis is induced mainly by certain bile salts, α-naphthylisocyanate, certain anabolic and contraceptive steroids, and manganese. This type of hepatic effect is different from those mentioned above in that those liver injuries do not result from cholestatic toxicants, the exception being manganese, which can also cause necrosis.

Chlorpromazine, erythromycin, phenytoin (diphenylhydantoin), and p-aminosalicylic acid appear to produce viral-like hepatitis through a type of hypersensitivity reaction. On the other hand, iproniazid, isoniazid, and hydrazine derivatives induce this effect perhaps through a metabolic abnormality.

Extensive lists of substances that induce various types of hepatic injury are provided by Zimmerman (1982).

TESTING PROCEDURES

Animals

The animals most commonly used are rats and mice. This is because of their ready availability, small size, low cost, ease in handling, and the relative abundance of toxicologic data. Furthermore, determinations of toxicities on the liver are often a part of short-term studies, which are often carried out in rats and mice. Sometimes dogs are used because of their greater susceptibility to a number of toxicants. Rhesus monkeys do not appear to be preferable to dogs because they are less susceptible and are more variable in their response (Gray, 1976).

Route of Administration

The chemical to be tested should be administered to the animals by the same route as the expected human exposure. However, in view of the relative difficulty in carrying out inhalation studies, it is interesting to note that the relative rankings of a number of halogenated hydrocarbons administered by parenteral route were similar to those obtained after administration by inhalation (Gehring, 1968).

Examinations

Gross Pathology The color and appearance can often indicate the nature of toxicity, such as fatty liver, or cirrhosis. The organ weight is often a very sensitive indicator of effect on the liver. Whereas an effect does not necessarily indicate toxicity, an increase in liver weight has been shown in certain cases to be the most sensitive criterion of toxicity. For instance, DA 1627 [α-methyl-α-morpholinoethyl)-1-naphthyl acetic acid] was found to significantly increase the absolute and relative liver weight at a dose level of 250 mg/kg/day without histologic changes. Fatty degeneration was observed in the animals dosed at a higher level, i.e., 1000 mg/kg (Bianchi et al., 1968).

Microscopic Examinations Light microscopy can detect a variety of histologic abnormalities, such as fatty change, necrosis, cirrhosis, hyperplastic nodules, neoplasia. Korsrud et al. (1972) found that CCl_4 produced histopathologic changes in the liver of rats at doses lower than those that induced changes in serum enzymes. Grice (1972) confirmed this finding with CCl_4 as well as with mercuric chloride, thioacetamide, and diethanolamine.

Electron microscopy appears to be as sensitive as light microscopy (Grice, 1972). It can detect changes in various subcellular structures. Observations of subcellular changes, along with biochemical findings, are often useful in delineating the mechanism of action of toxicants.

Biochemical Tests A number of serum enzymes have been used as indicators of hepatic injuries. These enzymes are released to the blood from the cytosol and subcellular organelles, such as mitochondria, lysosomes, and nuclei, as a result of hepatic injury. The most commonly used is SGPT (serum glutamic pyruvic transaminase). Its elevation is more marked than that of SGOT (serum glutamic oxaloacetic transaminase) with liver lesions. Sorbitol dehydrogenase is somewhat more sensitive to CCl_4, whereas isocitrate dehydrogenase and fructose-1-phosphate aldolase are about equally sensitive as SGPT. Alcohol dehydrogenase, 6-phosphogluconate dehydrogenase, and lactic and malic dehydrogenases are less sensitive (Korsrud et al., 1972). Other serum enzymes that have been used include alkaline phosphatase, 5-nucleotidase, leucine aminopeptidase, and arginase.

The liver is involved in the metabolism of carbohydrate, fat, and protein as well as in the formation of prothrombin and the excretion of bilirubin and certain foreign chemicals. It is also the major site of biotransformation of toxicants. Tests have thus been devised to determine these hepatic functions.

For example, the bilirubin level in the blood is an index of liver function, but it is relatively insensitive. The rate of excretion of BSP, a more sensitive indicator, is reduced when the liver is damaged. Clinically, the prolongation of prothrombin time, after excluding vitamin K deficiency, has been used in detecting acute hepatic lesions. A chemical may either potentiate or inhibit the pharmacologic and toxicologic actions of another by stimulating the hepatic microsomal enzymes (see Chapter 5). Measurements of barbiturate-induced sleeping time and the duration of zoxazolamine-induced paralysis have been used as indications of hepatic effects.

In addition, a number of biochemical tests can be performed on the liver tissue itself: (1) level of triglycerides, (2) activity of glucose-6-phosphatase, (3) level of microsomal conjugated dienes, resulting from peroxidation of microsomal lipids, (4) covalent binding of reactive metabolites to tissue macromolecules, (5) arylation or alkylation of purine and pyrimidine components of DNA and RNA (carcinogenicity), and (6) arylation or alkylation of other macromolecules (necrosis?).

IN VITRO TESTS

Isolated Perfused Liver

The rat liver has been isolated and perfused in the study of a wide range of effects on a variety of hepatotoxicants. For examples, the effects of CCl_4 on the transport and metabolism of triglycerides and fatty acids have been studied by Heimberg et al. (1962). Frazier and Kingsley (1976) reported on the transport of cadmium by the isolated liver to the bile. References to many other studies using this system have been provided by Zimmerman (1982).

Isolated Hepatocytes

Isolated rat and human hepatocytes, in suspension or in culture, have been used in a variety of biochemical studies. Freshly isolated hepatocytes are often used, but they can be maintained for only 2-6 hours. However, they can survive 1-5 days if kept in culture media. Normal hepatocytes have little or no mitotic activity. To study the effects on dividing liver cells, hepatocytes from very young animals or from liver tumors are used. The techniques involved in isolating and incubating these cells and in testing their viability are given by Klaassen and Stacey (1982).

The isolated hepatocytes can be used to determine the nature of various toxic effects:

1 Membrane damages can be detected microscopically or biochemically. Biochemical procedures include measuring the ability of the cells to take up cofactors (e.g., NADPH), polar dyes (e.g., trypan blue), and substrates (e.g., succinate) and leakage of cytoplasmic enzymes.

2 There may be changes in cellular macromolecules such as inhibition of protein and RNA synthesis and increased synthesis of DNA.

3 Other effects include alterations of intermediary metabolism and changes in the activity and growth of the hepatocytes.

EVALUATION

Nature of Toxicity

Certain effects on the liver, such as malignant neoplasm, are irreversible and serious. Necrosis may or may not be serious, depending on, for example, the extent of the effect. Local necrotic cells may be replaced by new cells through mitosis of adjacent hepatocytes. An accumulation of triglycerides per se is not necessarily indicative of damage. Under certain conditions the hepatocytes, with accumulated fat, function normally (Ingelfinger, 1971). The mortality rate in drug-induced cholestatic jaundice is less than 1%, whereas that in hepatocellular jaundice ranges from 10-50% (Zimmerman, 1982).

Quantitative Assessment

In general, microscopic changes are difficult to quantify. However, pathologic lesions can be graded according to their nature and extent (Grice, 1972; Zbinden,

1976). Quantitative stereology can be applied to light and electron microscopy. The tissue composition can be characterized in terms of volume, surface, and population density (de la Iglesia et al., 1982).

Biochemical findings can be readily analyzed statistically. The biochemical effects, when plotted against log dose, usually show linear dose-response relationship. This has been demonstrated, for example, in CCl_4-treated mice, with the following parameters: BSP retention, SGPT, bilirubinemia and triglycerides, glucose-6-phosphatase, and peroxidation (Plaa, 1976).

These dose-response relations can be used in comparing the relative toxicity of different chemicals. They can also be used in the assessment of the relative sensitivity of different parameters. For example, with a 10-fold increase in the dose of CCl_4, there was a 4- to 5-fold increase in SGPT, but only a 50% decrease in liver glucose-6-phosphatase (Plaa, 1976).

In assessing the severity of effect on the liver, it is important to bear in mind the differences between inducers (e.g., phenobarbital) and hepatotoxicants (e.g., CCl_4). With the former, the cellular responses generally include proliferation of the smooth membranes, increased drug-metabolizing activity, increased cytochrome P-450 content, and increased amounts of polyunsaturated acyl side-chains. On the other hand, hepatotoxicants disturb the structure of the endoplasmic reticulum, decrease the drug-metabolizing activity, decrease the cytochrome P-450 content, and increase the amount of saturated acyl side-chains (de la Iglesia et al., 1982).

REFERENCES

Bianchi, C., Bonardo, G., and Marazzi-Uberti, E. (1968) Toxicology of α-methyl-α-(2-morpholinoethyl)-1-naphthyl-acetic acid hydrochloride. *Toxicol. Appl. Pharmacol.* 12:331–336.

Boyer, J. L., Layden, T. J., and Hruban, Z. (1977) Mechanism of cholestasis—tauro-lithocholate alters canalicular membrane composition, structure and permeability. In: *Membrane Alterations as Basis of Liver Injury.* Eds. H. Popper, L. Biachi, and W. Reutter. Lancaster: MTP Press.

Bridges, J. W., Benford, D. J., and Hubbard, S. A. (1983) Mechanisms of toxic injury. *Ann. NY Acad. Sci.* 407:42–63.

de la Iglesia, F., Sturgess, J. M., and Feuer, G. (1982) New approaches for assessment of hepatotoxicity by means of quantitative functional-morphological interrelationship. In: *Toxicology of the Liver.* Eds. G. L. Plaa and W. R. Hewitt. New York: Raven Press.

Farber, E. (1975) Some fundamental aspects of liver injury. In: *Alcoholic Liver Injury.* Eds. J. M. Khanna, Y. Israel, and H. Kalant. Toronto: Addiction Research Foundation.

Frazier, J. M., and Kingsley, B. S. (1976) Kinetics of cadmium transport in the isolated perfused rat liver. *Toxicol. Appl. Pharmacol.* 38:583–593.

Gehring, P. J. (1968) Hepatotoxic potency of various chlorinated hydrocarbon vapors relative to their narcotic and lethal potencies in mice. *Toxicol. Appl. Pharmacol.* 13:287–298.

Gray, J. E. (1976) Assessment of hepatotoxic potential. *Environ. Health Perspect.* 15:47–54.

Grice, H. C. (1972) The changing role of pathology in modern safety evaluation. *CRC Crit. Rev. Toxicol.* 1:119–152.

Hartroft, W. S. (1975) On the etiology of alcoholic liver cirrhosis. In: *Alcoholic Liver Pathology.* Eds. J. M. Khanna, Y. Israel, and H. Kalant. Toronto: Addiction Research Foundation.

Heimberg, M., Weinstein, I., Dishmon, G., and Dunkerly, A. (1962) The action of carbon tetrachloride on the transport and metabolism of triglycerides and fatty acids by the isolated perfused rat liver and its relationship to the etiology of fatty liver. *J. Biol. Chem.* 237:3623–3627.

Hewitt, W. R., Miyajima, H., Côté, M. G., Hewitt, A., Cianflore, D. J., and Plaa, G. L. (1982) Dose-response relationships in 1,3-butanediol-induced potentiation of carbon tetrachloride toxicity. *Toxicol. Appl. Pharmacol.* 64:529–540.

Imai, K., and Hayashi, Y. (1970) Steroid-induced intrahepatic cholestasis in mice. *Jpn. J. Pharmacol.* 20:473–481.

Ingelfinger, F. J. (1971) Forward. In: *Regeneration of Liver and Kidney.* Eds. N. L. R. Butcher and R. A. Malt. Boston: Little, Brown.

Javitt, N. B., and Emerson, S. (1968) Effect of sodium taurolithocholate on bile flow and bile acid excretion. *J. Clin. Invest.* 47:1002–1014.

Klaassen, C. D., and Stacey, N. H. (1982) Use of isolated hepatocytes in toxicity assessment. In: *Toxicology of the Liver.* Eds. G. L. Plaa and W. R. Hewitt. New York: Raven Press.

Korsrud, G. O., Grice, H. C., and McLaughlan, J. M. (1972) Sensitivity of several serum enzymes in detecting carbon tetrachloride-induced liver damage in rats. *Toxicol. Appl. Pharmacol.* 22:474–483.

Kulkarni, A. P., and Hodgson, E. (1980) Hepatoxicity. In: *Introduction to Biochemical Toxicology.* Eds. E. Hodgson and F. E. Guthrie. New York: Elsevier.

Lieber, C. S., and DiCarli, L. M. (1976) Animal models of ethanol dependence of liver injury in rats and baboons. *Fed. Proc.* 35:1232–1236.

Mitchell, J. R., Snodgrass, W. R., and Gillette, J. R. (1976) The role of biotransformation in chemical-induced liver injury. *Environ. Health Perspect.* 15:27–38.

Newberne, P. M. (1982) Assessment of the hepatocarcinogenic potential of chemicals: Response of the liver. In: *Toxicology of the Liver.* Eds. G. L. Plaa and W. R. Hewitt. New York: Raven Press.

Plaa, G. L. (1976) Quantitative aspects in the assessment of liver injury. *Environ. Health Perspect.* 15:39–46.

Plaa, G. L. (1980) Toxic responses of the liver. In: *Casarett and Doull's Toxicology,* 2d ed. Eds. J. Doull, C. D. Klaassen, and M. O. Amdur. New York: Macmillan.

Plaa, G. L., and Priestly, B. G. (1976) Intrahepatic cholestasis induced by drugs and chemicals. *Pharmacol. Rev.* 28:207–273.

Recknagel, R. O., and Glende, E. A., Jr. (1973) Carbon tetrachloride hepato-toxicity: An example of lethal cleavage. *CRC Crit. Rev. Toxicol.* 2:263–297.

Recknagel, R. O., Glende, E. A., Waller, R. L., and Lowrey, K. (1982) Lipid peroxidation: Biochemistry, measurement, and significance in liver cell injury. In: *Toxicology of the Liver*. Eds. G. L. Plaa and W. R. Hewitt. New York: Raven Press.

Shah, H., Martman, S. P., and Weinhouse, S. (1979) Formation of carbonyl chloride in carbon tetrachloride metabolism by rat liver in vitro. *Cancer Res.* 39:3942–3947.

Smith, M. T., Loveridge, N., Wills, E. D., and Chayen, J. (1979) The distribution of glutathione in rat liver lobule. *Biochem. J.* 182:103–108.

Timbrell, J. A. (1982) Tissue lesions. In: *Principles of Biochemical Toxicology*. London: Taylor & Francis.

Wogan, C. N. (1976) The induction of liver cell cancer by chemicals. In: *Liver Cell Cancer*. Eds. H. M. Cameron, D. A. Linsell, and G. P. Warwick, Amsterdam: Elsevier.

Zbinden, G. (1976) The role of pathology in toxicology testing. In: *Progress in Toxicology*, Vol. 2. New York: Springer-Verlag.

Zimmerman, H. J. (1982) Chemiclal hepatic injury and its detection. In: *Toxicology of the Liver*. Eds. G. L. Plaa and W. R. Hewitt. New York: Raven Press.

ADDITIONAL READINGS

Heikel, T. A. J., and Lathe, G. H. (1970) The effect of oral contraceptives steroids on bile secretion and bilirubin Tm in rats. *Br. J. Pharmacol.* 38:593–600.

Slater, T. F. (1966) Necrogenic action of carbon tetrachloride in the rat: A speculative mechanism based on activation. *Nature* 209:36–40.

Chapter 14

Toxicology of the Kidney

INTRODUCTION

As noted in Chapter 2, the urine is the principal route by which most toxicants are excreted. For this reason, the kidney is a major target organ of toxic effects. To facilitate discussions on these effects, the renal structure and functions are briefly reviewed.

The predominant structures in the kidney are the nephrons, numbering approximately 1.3×10^6. Each nephron consists of a glomerulus and a series of tubules. (See Fig. 14-1.) The glomerulus is supplied with a high-pressure capilary system that produces an ultrafiltrate from the plasma. The filtrate collected in the Bowman's capsule flows through the proximal convoluted tubule, the loop of Henle, and the distal convoluted tubule and then drains through a collecting tubule into the renal pelvis for excretion as urine.

The major function of the kidney is to eliminate wastes resulting from normal metabolism and to excrete xenobiotics and their metabolites. These are effected through the production of urine, a process that also contributes to the maintenance of the homeostatic status of the body. In addition, it has several nonexcretory functions.

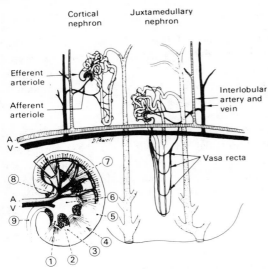

Figure 14-1 Lower left corner shows a sagittal section of a mammalian kidney. A and V refer to renal artery and vein, respectively. The various numbered parts are (1) minor calix, (2) fat in sinus, (3) renal column of Berlin, (4) medullary ray, (5) cortex, (6) pelvis, (7) interlobal artery, (8) major calix, (9) ureter. The remainder of the figure is an enlargement of a small segment of the sagittal section. It illustrates the two types of nephron (i.e., cortical and juxtamedullary), its various components, and the blood vessels—including the afferent and efferent arterioles entering and leaving the glomerulus and the vasa recta surrounding the loop of Henle. (From Tisher, 1981.)

The Production of Urine

A complex process is involved in the production of urine. It begins with the filtration in the glomeruli. In humans, approximately 180 liters of filtrate is formed per day. Since only 500–2500 ml of urine is excreted, some 99% of the filtered water is reabsorbed.

The reabsorption of water, through diffusion, takes place first at the proximal tubules, where Na^+ is actively reabsorbed. Further diffusion of water takes place at the descending limb of the loop of Henle to the hyperosmolar interstitium. The hyperosmolarity is produced by the active reabsorption of Cl^- (along with Na^+) at the ascending limb of the loop (Berndt, 1976). The spatial arrangement of the loops and the vasa recta provides an effective countercurrent multiplier mechanism.

Additional water is removed from the filtrate in the distal and the collecting tubules as Na^+ is actively reabsorbed. However, the extent of the removal of water from these tubules depends on the activity of antidiuretic hormone (ADH). ADH reduces the urine volume by increasing the permeability of these structures to water.

Tubular Resorption and Secretion

As the glomerular capillaries have larger pores (40 Å), substances with molecular weights under 60,000 are filtered into Bowman's capsules. Some of the filtered substances such as glucose and amino acids, which are vital to the body, are reabsorbed by the tubules. On the other hand, ammonia (NH_3), a metabolic waste of amino acids, diffuses through the cells to the filtrate, where it reacts with H^+ to form NH_4^+, which is excreted.

To facilitate the passive reabsorption of water and to maintain the homeostasis, various electrolytes in the glomerular filtrate are reabsorbed nearly completely or to a great extent. The reabsorption of Na^+ at the distal and collecting tubules is regulated by the mineralocorticoids, that of phosphorus by the parathyroid hormone and that of bicarbonate (HCO_3^-) by the acid-base balance. In addition, K^+ and H^+ are secreted by the tubules.

Nonexcretory Functions

The kidney possesses other functions, such as the regulation of blood pressure and volume. This is mediated through the renin-angiotensin-aldosterone system. Renin, a proteolytic enzyme, is formed in the cells of the juxtaglomerular apparatus and catalyzes the conversion of a plasma angiotensin prohormone to angiotensin I. The latter, a decapeptide, is converted in the lung to angiotensin II by an enzyme that removes a dipeptide from the C-terminal end.

A renal erythropoietic factor (REF) also acts on a plasma protein to form erythropoietin, which increases the production of normoblasts and the synthesis of hemoglobin. Renal prostaglandins are produced in the interstitial cells in the medulla and appear to have the capability of regulating renal blood flow and the excretion of Na^+ and urine. The kidney is also involved in the conversion of the relatively inactive 25-hydroxy-vitamin D_3 to the active 1,25-dihydroxy-vitamin D_3.

SITE AND TYPE OF TOXICITY

All parts of the nephron are potentially subject to the detrimental effects of toxicants. The effects range in severity from one or more biochemical aberrations to cell death, and they can manifest as minor alterations of renal function or complete renal failure.

Glomeruli

Nephrotoxins, e.g., puromycin, can increase the permeability of the glomerulus to proteins such as albumin. This has been attributed to an alteration in the electrical charge of glomerular basement membrane (Brenner et al., 1977).

Proximal Tubules

Because of their active absorptive and secretory activities, the proximal tubules often have higher concentrations of toxicants and are thus often the site of toxic effects. Heavy metals, such as mercury, chromium, cadmium, and lead, can alter the functions of the tubules, characterized by glucosuria, aminoaciduria, and polyuria. After higher doses, they cause cell death. The straight portion (pars recta) of the proximal tubules appears more susceptible than the convoluted portion to the toxicity of mercury (Phillips et al., 1977). This conslusion is based on the observation that at low doses, the p-aminohippuric acid (PAH) secretion is reduced, whereas glucosuria develops only at somewhat higher doses. PAH is secreted at the pars recta and glucose is reabsorbed in the proximal convoluted tubules. In addition to PAH (an organic anion), organic cations, such as tetraethylammonium (TEA) and N-methylnicotinamide (NMN), are also actively secreted.

Many antibiotics are also secreted by the proximal tubules and can induce alterations in the tubular functions. Streptomycin, neomycin, kanamycin, cephaloridine, amphotericin B, and the tetracyclines have all been reported to affect the functions of the proximal tubules (Hook, 1980).

Halogenated hydrocarbons such as carbon tetrachloride and chloroform are essentially hepatoxic, but in certain animal species they may also exert toxic effects on the kidney, especially on the proximal tubules, as reflected in functional changes. At higher doses, however, morphologic changes may be produced in other parts of the nephron.

Other Sites

The distal tubules may be affected by nephrotoxins such as amphotericin B, resulting in decreased acidification of the urine, since one of the functions of these tubules is the secretion of H^+.

The nephrotoxicity of heavy metals may result partly from the vasoconstriction, possibly involving renal prostaglandins (Hook, 1980).

Methoxyflurane, an anesthetic, is known to be nephrotoxic in humans, causing *high-output* renal failure. Mazze (1976) suggested that the chemical interferes with the reabsorption of Na^+ and water at the proximal tubules, resulting in an overloading of the distal parts of the nephron and in an interference of their functions. It also inhibits the enzyme systems involved in the sodium (or chloride) pumping in the ascending limb of the loop of Henle, thus reducing the interstitial osmolarity. As a result, there is a decreased water resorption. Additionally, damages to the collecting tubules render them insensitive to ADH, which further reduces water resorption.

Analgesic mixtures containing aspirin and phenacetin can cause chronic renal failure, with the toxic effects located predominantly in the medulla. The effects might be a result of a basoconstriction of the vasa recta due to an inhibition of the synthesis of vasodilator prostaglandin (Nanra and Kincaid-Smith, 1974). Other types of toxicity include renal carcinogenicity of DMN (dimethylnitrosamine), and tubular blockade induced by the metabolites of sulfapyridine (acetylsulfapyridine) and glycols (oxalic acid).

Penicillins and sulfonamides have been reported to cause inflammatory interstitial nephritis in humans. An immunologic mechanism has been suggested as responsible for this toxicity (Appel and Neu, 1977).

TESTING PROCEDURE

Functional and morphologic examinations of the kidney are routinely carried out as an integral part of short-term and long-term toxicity studies. The types of examinations involved are described in Chapters 6 and 8, and are further elaborated in this section.

In studies designed specifically for nephrotoxicity, dogs, rabbits, and rats are the commonly used animals. Examinations of the kidney functions may be done in a number of ways.

Urinalysis

Proteinuria Because of the size of their molecules, a very small amount of proteins of low molecular weight pass through the glomerular filter. The low molecular weight proteins are readily reabsorbed by the proximal tubules. The occurrence of large amounts of protein in the urine is thus an indication of a loss of integrity of glomeruli. It is to be noted that normal rat urine may contain some protein. A critical comparison of the treated animals with the controls is therefore important.

Glycosuria Glucose in the glomerular filtrate is completely reabsorbed in the tubules, provided the amount of glucose to be reabsorbed does not exceed the *transport maximum* (Tm). Glycosuria in the absence of hyperglycemia thus indicates tubular dysfunction.

Urine Volume and Osmolarity These two values are usually inversely related and are useful indicators of renal function in *concentration test*, wherein water is withheld from the animal, and also in *dilution test*, wherein a large amount of water is given to the animal. The osmolarity can be estimated from the specific gravity, but the freezing point of urine provides a more accurate measurement. A toxicant may cause high-output renal failure as noted above. On the other hand, it may cause oliguria or even anuria, resulting from tubular injury, with concomitant interstitial edema and intraluminal pigment or debris.

Acidifying Capacity This can be assessed from urine pH, titratable acids, and NH_4^+. This capacity is reduced when there is distal tubular dysfunction.

Enzymes Enzymes such as maltase in urine may indicate destruction of proximal tubules. Lysozyme level in urine is greatly increased following intoxication with chromium, but only moderately so after mercury poisoning. Urine alkaline phosphatase, on the other hand, may be renal or hepatic in origin. Plummer (1981) suggests that the levels of urinary enzymes not only are useful indicators of renal damage but also indicate the subcellular site of origin. For example, alkaline phosphatase is located in endoplasmic reticulum, glutamate dehydrogenase in mitochondria, and lactate dehydrogenase in cytoplasm. In general, urinary enzymes are more useful in acute nephrotoxic conditions.

Proteins High molecular weight proteins are normally not filtered through the glomeruli. Their appearance in urine therefore indicates glomerular damage. On the other hand, low molecular weight proteins do pass through the glomerular filter, but they are reabsorbed by the proximal tubules. If this tubular function is impaired, such proteins will appear in the urine, e.g., in cadmium poisoning.

Blood Analysis

Blood Urea Nitrogen (BUN) Blood urea nitrogen is derived from normal metabolism of protein and is excreted in the urine. Elevated BUN usually indicates glomerular damage. However, its level can also be affected by poor nutrition and hepatotoxicity, which are common effects of many toxicants.

Creatinine Creatinine is a metabolite of creatine and is excreted completely in the urine via glomerular filtration. An elevation of its level in the blood is thus an indication of impaired kidney function. Furthermore, data on its level in blood and its amounts in urine can be used to estimate the glomerular filtration rate. One drawback with this procedure is the fact that some creatinine is secreted by the tubules.

Special Tests

Glomerular Filtration Rate (GFR) The glomerular filtration rate can be more accurately determined by the clearance of inulin, a polysaccharide. It is diffused into the glomerular filtrate and is neither reabsorbed nor secreted by the tubules.

Renal Clearance This is the volume of plasma that is completely cleared of a substance in a unit of time. The renal clearance of p-aminohippuric acid (PAH) exceeds that of inulin because it is not only filtered through the glomeruli but also secreted by the tubules. A reduction of PAH elimination without a concomitant decrease of GFR indicates tubular dysfunction. PAH is nearly completely (up to 90%) removed from the blood in one passage. The rate of its clearance is therefore useful in determining the effective renal plasma flow (ERPF). The renal blood flow can also be determined by the use of radiolabeled microspheres or an electromagnetic flowmeter.

PSP Excretion Test The rate of excretion of phenolsulfonphthlein is related to renal blood flow. It is, therefore, often used in the assessment of renal function. However, a reduced secretion rate can also result from cardiovascular diseases.

Morphologic Examinations

Gross Examination The organ weight of the kidney per se or in terms of body weight of the animal, as a rule, is routinely determined at the end of short-term and long-term toxicity studies. Alterations in the organ weight, when compared to the controls, often suggest kidney lesions. A number of other pathologic lesions can also be detected on gross examination.

Light Microscopy Histopathologic examinations can reveal the site, extent, and morphologic nature of renal lesions. Sharrat and Frazer (1963) found that the histopathologic examinations were more sensitive than the functional tests used by the authors in assessing 15 acute and chronic glomerular or tubular injuries. However, some of the newer functional tests appear more sensitive (see In Vitro Studies section to follow).

Electron Microscopy This procedure is useful in assessing ultrastructural changes in the cells, such as mitochondria, other organelles, basement membranes, and brush border. For example, prolonged exposure to methyl mercury increased the volume density of mitochondria and lysosomes. Concomitantly, there were changes in various enzyme activities, the most notable of which was the marked increase in the specific activity of δ-aminolevulinic acid synthetase (Fowler, 1980). Trump and his co-workers classified control and renal ultrastructural changes according to the apparent severity into five groups (see Berndt, 1976a). Further work, however, is needed to elucidate the significance of these various changes in terms of renal function.

In Vitro Studies

Kidney Slices Tissue slices provide a useful tool for the study of renal tubular function. In spite of the relatively artificial conditions imposed by in vitro studies, Berndt (1976b) compiled data demonstrating that the in vitro uptakes of various organic acids, bases, sugars, amino acids, and inorganic electrolytes were essentially identical to those under in vivo conditions.

A toxicant to be studied can be added to the medium in which the slices are immersed, or it can be administered to the animal prior to the removal of the kidney for the preparation of the slices. For example, Koschier and Berndt (1976) reported that renal slices from animals pretreated with 2,4,5-trichloro-phenoxyacetic acid (2,4,5-T) showed impaired renal transport of 2,4,5-T, 2,4-dichlorophenoxyacetic acid (2,4-D), and TEA in the absence of morphologic changes. A description of the method used in studying nephrotoxins on kidney slices and the results obtained thereof as well as extensive literature citations are provided by Kacew and Hirsch (1982).

Perfused Renal Tubules Various sections of the renal tubules of the rabbit have been isolated and their transport functions studied. In addition, other species of animals have been used; these include the mouse, rat, hamster, snake, flounder, frog, salamander, and humans. Schafer (1981) described the technique and outlined the pros and cons of this procedure.

Isolated Nephrons Endou et al. (1983) isolated nephrons from rat kidney after perfusing it with 0.1% collagenase to facilitate the dissection. They found cytochrome P-450 existent only in the proximal tubules, the straight portion containing more than the convoluted portion. Furthermore, the enzyme in these two portions of the tubule differ in their responses to 3-methylcholanthrene and starvation.

EVALUATION

Nature of Toxicity

The kidney has a remarkable compensatory capability. Even after appreciable changes in renal functions and morphology, the kidney may compensate and regain normal functions. Therefore, it is important to perform tests at repeated and appropriate time intervals.

Nephrotoxins can exert adverse effects on various parts of the kidney, resulting in alterations of different functions. A variety of tests should therefore be performed. The most sensitive and reliable tests appear to vary depending on the nature of the nephrotoxin as well as the experimental conditions, e.g., animal species, duration of exposure. In an article, Luwe (1981) concluded from his studies that in vitro accumulation of organic ions (e.g., PAH, TEA), urinary concentrating ability, and kidney weight were the most sensitive and consistent indicators of nephrotoxicity. Standard urinalysis, serum analyses, qualitative enzymuria, and histopathologic changes were less sensitive and less consistent. Goldstein et al. (1981) observed that urine osmolarity was the most sensitive indicator of the nephrotoxicity of a platinum complex, whereas GFR and ERPF were affected only later and at higher doses.

In assessing the renal effects of a toxicant, extrarenal factors that might affect the blood volume or blood pressure should be taken into account, since they may indirectly impair renal functions. Furthermore, kidney diseases, such as those associated with aging, may be prevalent and should also be considered (Cotchin and Roe, 1967).

Quantitative Assessment

In general, morphologic changes are difficult to quantify. However, criteria for grading the microscopic changes have been suggested by Zbinden (1976) and Trump (1970).

On the other hand, biochemical and functional tests usually yield data that can be statistically analyzed readily. Since nephrotoxins may affect several renal functions differently, quantitative comparison of relative toxicity should be done with caution.

REFERENCES

Appel, G. B., and Neu, H. C. (1977) The nephrotoxicity of antimicrobial agents (parts 1 and 2). *N. Engl. J. Med.* 296:663–670, 722–728.

Berndt, W. O. (1976a) Renal function tests: What do they mean? A review of renal anatomy, biochemistry, and physiology. *Environ. Health Perspect.* 15:55–71.

Berndt, W. O. (1976b) Use of tissue slice technique for evaluation of renal transport processes. *Environ. Health Perspect.* 15:73–88.

Brenner, B. M., Bohrer, M. P., Baglis, C., and Deen, W. M. (1977) Determinants of glomerular permselectivity: Insights derived from observations in vivo. *Kidney Int.* 12:229–257.

Cotchin, E., and Roe, F. J. C. (1967) *Pathology of Laboratory Rats and Mice.* Oxford: Blackwell Scientific.

Endou, H., Koseki, C., and Sakai, F. (1983) Effects of 3-methylcholanthrene and starvation on intranephron distribution of cytochrome P-450. *Toxicol. Lett.* 18(Suppl. 1):110.

Fowler, B. A. (1980) Ultrastructural morphometric/biochemical assessment of cellular toxicity. In: *The Scientific Basis of Toxicity Assessment.* Ed. P. R. Witschi. Amsterdam: Elsevier/North Holland.

Goldstein, R. S., Noordwier, B., Bond, J. T., Hook, J. B., and Mayor, G. H. (1981) cis-Dichlorodiammineplatinum nephrotoxicity: Time course and dose response of renal functional impairment. *Toxicol. Appl. Pharmacol.* 60:163–175.

Hook, J. B. (1980) Toxic responses of the kidney. In: *Casarett and Doull's Toxicology.* Eds. J. Doull, C. D. Klaassen, and M. O. Amdur. New York: Macmillan.

Kacew, S., and Hirsch, G. H. (1982) Evaluation of nephrotoxicity of various compounds by means of in vitro techniques and comparison to in vivo methods. In: *Toxicology of the Kidney.* Eds. J. B. Hook. New York: Raven Press.

Kluwe, W. M. (1981) Renal function tests as indicators of kidney injury in subacute toxicity studies. *Toxicol. Appl. Pharmacol.* 57:414–424.

Koschier, E. F., and Berndt, W. O. (1976) In vitro uptake of organic ions by renal cortical tissue of rats treated acutely with 2,4,5-trichlorophenoxy-acetic acids. *Toxicol. Appl. Pharmacol.* 35:355–364.

Mazze, R. I. (1976) Methoxyflurane nephropathy. *Environ. Health Perspect.* 15:111–120.

Nanra, R. S., and Kincaid-Smith, P. (1972) Pathology, etiology and pathogenesis of analgesic nephropathy. *Aust. N.Z. J. Med.* 4:602–603.

Phillips, R., et al. (1977) Assessment of mercuric chloride-induced nephrotoxicity by *p*-aminohippuric acid uptake and the activity of four gluconeogenic enzymes in rat renal cortex. *Toxicol. Appl. Pharmacol.* 41:407–422.

Plummer, D. T. (1981) Urinary enzyme in drug toxicity. In: *Testing for Toxicity*. Ed. J. W. Gorrod. London: Taylor & Franics.

Schafer, J. A. (1981) Transport studies in isolated perfused renal tubules. *Fed. Proc.* 40:2450–2459.

Sharratt, M., and Frazer, A. C. (1963) The sensitivity of function tests in detecting renal damage in the rat. *Toxicol. Apply. Pharmacol.* 5:36–48.

Tisher (1981) In: *The Kidney*, 2d ed., p. 5. Eds. B. M. Brenner and F. C. Rector. Philadelphia: Saunders.

Trump, B. F. (1970) Ion movements in cell injury. In: *Proceedings of the 4th International Congress of Nephrology*, Vol. 1.S, p. 88. Basel: Karger.

Zbinden, G. (1976) *Progress in Toxicology, Vol. 2.* New York: Springer-Verlag.

Chapter 15

Toxicology of the Skin

GENERAL CONSIDERATIONS

The body of humans, as well as that of animal, is almost entirely covered by skin. As a result, it is exposed to a variety of chemicals such as cosmetics, household products, topical medication, and industrial pollutants, especially in certain workplaces. Dermal exposure to chemicals can result in various types of lesions. Furthermore, skin lesions may follow systematic exposure to chemicals.

The skin consists of the epidermis and the dermis, which rests over the subcutaneous tissue (Fig. 15-1). The epidermis is relatively thin, averaging 0.1–0.2 mm in thickness, whereas the dermis is about 2 mm thick. These two layers are separated by a basement membrane.

The epidermis in turn consists of a basal cell layer (stratum germinativum), which provides the other layers with new cells. These new cells become prickle cells (stratum spinosum) and, later, the granular cells (stratum granulosum). The nuclei in these cells disintegrate and dissolve. In addition, these cells produce keratohydrin, which later becomes keratin in the outermost stratum

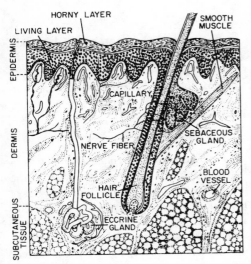

Figure 15-1 Cross section of the skin showing the two major layers of epidermis and dermis, and the various structures in the dermis. (From *The Skin,* by W. M. Montagna. Copyright © 1965 by Scientific American, Inc. All rights reserved.)

corneum. This layer is gradually shed. This development process takes about 4 weeks. The epidermis also contains melanocytes, which produce pigments; the Langerhans cells, which act as macrophages; and lymphocytes. The latter two types of cells are involved in immune responses. The epidermis thus forms an important protective cover of the body.

The dermis is mainly composed of collagen and elastin, which are important structures for the support of the skin. In this layer, there are several types of cells, the most abundant being the fibroblasts, which are involved in the biosynthesis of the fibrous proteins and ground substances such as hyaluronic acid, chondroitin sulfates, and mucopolysaccharides. The other types of cells include fat cells, macrophages, histiocytes, and mast cells. Underneath the dermis is the subcutaneous tissue.

There are, in addition, a number of other structures. These include the hair follicles, sweat glands, sebaceous glands, small blood vessels, and neural elements, including Meissner's corpuscles.

The possibility of systemic toxicity following dermal exposure to toxicants is discussed in Chapter 2. A good review of the systemic toxicity of a number of pesticides, industrial chemicals, and medications after cutaneous absorption is available (Birmingham, 1977).

TYPES OF TOXIC EFFECTS

A variety of effects can result from dermal exposure to toxicants. Most of the effects involve the skin itself, but some of them affect its appendages—hair, sebaceous glands, and sweat glands.

Primary Irritation

Irritation is a reaction of the skin to chemicals such as strong alkalis, acids, solvents, soaps, and detergents. It ranges in severity from hyperemia, edema, and vesiculation to ulceration (corrosion). Primary irritations occur at the site of contact and, in general, on the first contact. It is thus different from sensitization.

Sensitization Reaction

The skin may show little or no reaction on contact with a chemical. However, a reaction or a more severe reaction occurs after a subsequent exposure to the chemical. This delayed reaction, with a latent period ranging from a few days to years, apparently involves a complex immune mechanism. After penetration through the epidermis, the toxicant forms a covalent bond with certain proteins. Aoki et al. (1969) detected 15 different types of antigenic proteins in the skin besides the serum proteins, which may also form conjugates with the hapten. Despite the various types of autologous proteins, their conjugates with a particular hapten probably have the same immunogenicity (Polak, 1977).

Sensitization reactions often result from topical medications such as antibiotics, antihistamines, local anesthetics, antiseptics, and stabilizers (e.g., ethylenediamine). Other substances include plants (e.g., poison ivy), metal compounds, dyes, cosmetics, and industrial agents.

Phototoxicity and Photoallergy

These two types of skin reaction are similar in that both are light-induced and may follow either systemic administration or topical application of the offending chemical. However, photoallergy involves immune reactions, whereas phototoxicity does not. This and other differences have been summarized by Harber and Baer (1972) (Table 15-1).

Phototoxicity is much more common than photoallergy. The commonly reported phototoxic chemicals in humans, according to Harber and Shalita (1977), are sulfonamides, sulfonylureas, chlorothiazides, phenothiazines, demeclocycline, psoralens, coal tar, anthracene, pyridine, acridine, and phenanthrene. The skin reaction consists of a delayed erythema, followed by hyperpigmentation and desquamation.

The commonly reported photoallergic chemicals, according to Harber and Shalita (1977), are halogenated salicylanilides and related compounds, sulfonamides, griseofulyin, fentichlor [2,2'-thiobis(4-chlorophenol)], multifungin, promethazine, Blankophores, cyclamates, thiazides, tolbutamide, chlorpropamide, chlorpromazine, chlordiazepoxide, and triacetyldiphenolisatin. Many compounds are therefore both phototoxic and photoallergic. Clinically, photoallergy usually manifests as delayed papules and eczema, but it may also appear

Table 15-1   Comparison of Phototoxic and Photoallergic Reactions

Reaction	Phototoxic	Photoallergic
Reaction possible on first exposure	Yes	No
Incubation period necessary first exposure	No	Yes
Chemical alteration of photosensitizer	No	Yes
Covalent binding with carrier	No	Yes
Clinical changes	Usually like sunburn	Varied morphology
Flares at distant previously involved sites possible	No	Yes
Persistent light reaction can develop	No	Yes
Cross-reactions to structurally related agents	Infrequent	Frequent
Broadening of cross-reactions following repeated photopatch testing	No	Possible
Concentration of drug necessary for reaction	High	Low
Incidence	Usually relatively high (theoretically 100%)	Usually very low (but theoretically could reach 100%)
Action spectrum	Usually similar to absorption	Usually higher wavelength than absorption spectrum
Passive transfer	No	Possible
Lymphocyte stimulation test	No	Possible
Macrophage migration inhibition test	No	Possible

Source: Harber and Baer, 1972.

as immediate urticarial reaction. Histologically it is characterized by a dense perivascular round cell infiltrate in the dermis. The delayed reactions are cell-mediated immune response, whereas the immediate reaction is probably antibody-mediated (Epstein, 1977).

The most biologically active rays that cause erythema and pigmentation are in the shorter ultraviolet range, i.e., wavelengths below 320 nm. The sunlight ranges from 290 nm upwards, but the UV rays emitted by artificial light sources may be shorter. However, the longer UV rays (320–400 nm) are less erythrogenic per se but are responsible for both phototoxic and photoallergic reactions to chemicals (see p. 213).

Contact Urticaria

This is a special type of reaction, involving mainly the skin in contact with the offending agent, but sometimes there are also systemic effects. The systemic effects include generalized urticarial and anaphylactoid reactions. Odom and

Maibach (1977) listed a variety of chemicals and a few physical agents that reportedly elicit such phenomena and classified the mechanisms under three categories.

Nonimmunologic Mechanism The local urticaria appears quickly and is probably induced by the released histamine, bradykinin, slow reacting substance A (SRS-A), and certain other vasoactive substances. This type of reaction occurs after topical application of, for example, dimethyl sulfoxide, Trafuryl (tetra-hydrofurfuryl ester of nicotinic acid), and cobalt chloride solution.

Immunologic Mechanism This mechanism is involved in the appearance of local urticaria as well as generalized urticaria and anaphylactoid reactions. The incriminated agents include chemicals such as monoamylamine, mechloretha-mine hydrochloride, diethyltoluamide, tetanus antitoxin, bacitracin, penicillin, and streptomycin. Potato has also been reported to cause this phenomenon among susceptible housewives (Pearson, 1966). Passive transfer test (see Testing Procedures Section) is positive among many of the affected individuals.

Uncertain Mechanisms Ammonium persulfate, a powerful oxidizing agent, is an active ingredient in hair bleach. Brubaker (1972) and others have reported on this chemical as causing generalized erythema, urticaria, and shock.

Cutaneous Cancer

It has been known for over two centuries that soots can cause skin cancer. More recent studies confirm that soots and related substances, e.g., coal tars, creosote oils, shale oils, and cutting oil, cause cancers of the skin and other sites in animals and humans. In addition, arsenic and certain arsenic compounds have been reported to be associated with skin cancer in humans (see IARC, 1979).

A number of polycyclic aromatic hydrocarbons (e.g., benzo[a]pyrene), and heterocyclic compounds (e.g., benz[c]acridine) are known to induce skin cancer after topical applications on animals (IARC, 1973).

Effects on Epidermal Adnexa

Hair Loss of hair may result from various antimitotic agents used in cancer chemotherapy. These agents affect the anagen phase of hair growth. The affected hair starts to shed after about 2 weeks of therapy, but hair growth resumes about 2 months after the suspension of therapy.

A number of other medications are known to cause hair loss by converting hair follicles in anagen phase to telogen phase. In such cases, hair shedding generally starts 2-4 months after therapy. The medications involved in this type of hair loss include oral contraceptives, anticoagulants, propranolol, and triparanol. Agents causing hair loss of unknown mechanism include antithyroid drugs and excessive intake of vitamin A.

Sebaceous Glands These glands secrete lipid through expulsion of their lipid-laden cells and are therefore known as *holocrine*. Their activity is hormone-dependent. For example, androgens stimulate and estrogens inhibit the excretion. Adrenocortical steroids and thyroid hormones also have some stimulatory activity. The effects of the pituitary are complex, acting both directly and indirectly via other endocrine organs.

A number of chlorinated aromatic hydrocarbons can cause various skin lesions, including chloracne. The severity of acne varies, but it has been confined mainly to occupational workers. Notable exceptions were the outbreaks in Japan among individuals after their consumption of a batch of rice oil contaminated with polychlorinated biphenyls (PCB) (WHO, 1976) and in Seveso, Italy, among residents near a factory that accidentally released a large amount of TCDD (2,3,7,8-tetrachlorodibenzo-*p*-dioxin) (Pocchiari, 1980).

Sweat Glands Sweating serves useful physiologic functions such as regulation of body temperature. Blockage of the sweat ducts, a disorder known as miliaria, may occur after topical application of 95% phenol and chloroform (Shelley and Horvath, 1950). Systematically, atabrine can cause anhidrosis. A number of antimitotic agents and overdosage with CNS depressants can cause necrosis of the sweat glands (Reller and Luedders, 1977).

TESTING PROCEDURES

For most effects on skin, the test animal of choice is the albino rabbit, although albino guinea pigs, white mice, and others are also used.

Primary Irritation

This effect is in generaly measured by a patch test on the skin of rabbits (Draize, 1959). A small amount (0.5 g or 0.5 ml) of the chemical to be tested is introduced under a 1 square inch gauze pad that is placed over a shaved part of the skin. The pad is suitably fastened over the animal for 24 hours. At the end of this period, the pad is removed and the skin reaction is graded according to the extent of (1) erythema and eschar formation and (2) edema formation. The skin reaction is read again at the end of 72 hours. The same test is done on other rabbits, except that the skin has been abraded. The 24- and 72-hour readings from both groups are added to obtain the *primary irritation index*. The test procedure, grading of skin reaction, and the interpretation of the grading are given in Appendix 15-1.

There are a number of modified skin irritation tests based on the Draize procedure. The modifications involve the animal species used, amount of test material applied, repetitive applications, and types of examinations, e.g., histologic (Hood, 1977; McCreesh and Steinberg, 1977).

Sensitization Reaction

The procedure described by Draize (1959) calls for the use of guinea pigs that are given the chemical by 10 repeated intradermal injections on one flank and a challenging dose on the other flank after a 10- to 14-day resting period. A greater reaction after the challenging dose, in comparison with that after the sensitizing doses, indicates sensitization.

The Draize test is generally considered insufficiently sensitive to identify allergic potential. Furthermore, the intradermal injection is considered inappropriate to assess the safety of chemicals to be applied on the surface of the skin. A number of modifications have thus been proposed. The procedures in detail have been compiled by Klecak (1977). Highlights of some of them are given here.

Freund Complete Adjuvant Test This test involves the use of Freund adjuvant in order to enhance the sensitivity. Furthermore, in challenging the treated animals, four concentrations of the chemical are given, thus providing a basis for quantitative estimation. However, as in the Draize test, the test material is given by intradermal injection.

Epicutaneous Methods One of these methods (Buehler test) stipulates that the test substance, after dilution, be applied topically to the skin and held in place for 6 hours by means of an occlusive patch for the induction and challenge. In the other, the *open epicutaneous test*, the undiluted compound and/or its progressive dilutions are applied to the skin, which remains uncovered. With the former method, only three induction doses are applied at weekly intervals, whereas the latter method calls for 21 daily applications.

Intradermal and Epicutaneous Applications According to the maximization test, the guinea pigs are given intradermally on day 0 the test substance with and without Freund complete adjuvant. On day 7 the substance is applied at the same site occlusively. Two weeks later, the test substance is applied topically over the pretreated areas in these animals. Different concentrations of the agent are used in the challenge. With split-adjuvant technique, the test material is applied occlusively three times and injected intradermally once. The challenging dose is applied occlusively.

The validity of the results from these tests has been checked against human experience. Human experience is obtained either in patch tests or in a controlled population. In the latter case, the substance is widely distributed to the target population for use as directed. Their skin reactions are examined and evaluated. A patch test usually involves 100 males and 100 females, covering a wide age range. The test material (0.5 ml or 0.5 g) is applied by patch to an area on the arm or back. The skin reaction is examined on the following day after the removal of the patch.

Phototoxicity and Photoallergy

Phototoxicity appears to be more readily demonstrable in the hairless mouse, the rabbit, and the guinea pig. The substance to be tested may be administered topically or by a systemic route. The reaction of the skin to nonerythrogenic light (wavelength greater than 320 nm) is then determined. Significant erythema, compared to controls, indicates phototoxicity.

For the detection of photoallergy, albino guinea pigs are especially useful. The procedure involves, in principle, an induction of photosensitization by repeatedly applying a small amount of the chemical on a shaved and depilated area of the skin and exposing that area to appropriate UV rays. After a 3-week interval, the guinea pigs are exposed to the chemical and the UV rays to elicit photoallergy. Details of the procedure are given by Harber and Shalita (1977).

Contact Urticaria

A number of animal models have been proposed based on the procedure devised by Jacobs (1940). Using the patch test on the flank and nipples of guinea pigs, Hunziker (1977) described the gross and histologic changes produced by a variety of chemicals. Some of these, e.g., dinitrochlorobenzene, produced reactions after one application, whereas others, e.g., *p*-nitrosodimethylaniline, required several applications. Recently, a test using guinea pig ears has been found satisfactory in screening human contact urticarigenic substances (Lahti and Maibach, 1984).

The open patch test can be applied to human volunteers or to patients suspected of being susceptible to the chemical. In the latter case, all necessary resuscitation equipment and personnel should be available to respond to anaphylactoid reaction.

Any immunologic involvement can be demonstrated by the passive transfer test, in which 0.1 ml fresh serum from the patient is injected intradermally into the forearm of a volunteer and challenged 24 hours later by applying the suspect chemical to the injection site.

Cutaneous Cancer

The procedure involves topical application of the substance on a shaved area of the skin. The substance per se, if a liquid, is applied directly. Otherwise, it is dissolved or suspended in a suitable vehicle. The skin painting is usually done once a week or more frequently. The commonly used animal is the mouse. It is advisable to include a vehicle control group as well as a positive control group, which is treated with a known skin carcinogen such as benzo[a]pyrene.

Others

Hair Loss   This is usually tested in guinea pigs. The chemical is administered by the same route as that to be encountered in human exposure conditions. A vehicle control group is included to assist in the interpretation of the results. There may be noticeable diffuse or spotty loss of hair. Otherwise, the pluck test and pull test will be necessary (Reeves and Maibach, 1977).

Acne   Kligman and Katz (1968) described a test according to which the test material is inserted in the external ear canal of rabbits. Positive reactions are marked by thickened mounds on the follicles, caused by distention with horny materials.

EVALUATION

Although various tests for primary irritation and sensitization reaction have been in use for many years, their reliability and reproducibility have been questioned. An extensive intralaboratory and interlaboratory study showed that the range of skin irritation scores was relatively small in some laboratories and large in others (Weil and Scala, 1972). The authors suggested that courses be conducted for the technicians involved.

The validity of these tests has been evaluated in a number of studies comparing the skin reaction to chemicals in humans and various animals. For example, Carter and Griffith (1965) and Phillips et al. (1972) reported poor agreement between human and rabbit patch test. Roudabush et al. (1965) showed that for a number of chemicals the guinea pig was a suitable alternative to the rabbit. More recently, Nixon et al. (1975) and Griffith and Buehler (1977) found the rabbit to be generally more susceptible than the guinea pig and humans, and the use of these two species is more reliable in predicting human reactions. Furthermore, the use of abraded skin did not enhance the value of the animal tests.

The various sensitization tests in guinea pigs and the human patch test yielded comparable results to a variety of chemicals (Magnusson and Kligman, 1977). However, these tests appear to be more likely to yield false-positive results than false-negatives, compared to use experience in humans. One contributing factor may be the sensitizing activity of ethanol under the test conditions in guinea pigs and humans, but nonexistent in actual use (Griffith and Buehler, 1977).

There is less information comparing results from the various tests in animals and human experience with respect to the other types of dermal effects. However, the available information indicates that they are useful as screening procedures.

The testing procedures outlined in the previous section have been widely used, despite certain deficiencies. Seeking to improve on them, Middleton (1981) has proposed the following new approaches, which are designed to measure more specific biologic and biochemical events:

1   Effects of chemicals on stratum corneum barrier function as determined by transdermal water loss and electrical conductance

2   Alterations in the normal differentiation pattern of epidermis, which are demonstrable by measuring, in different layers, the contents of phospholipids, keratin, and a histidine-rich protein

3   Changes in epidermal cell proliferation as shown by the mitotic index among basal cells and the rate of DNA synthesis

4   Changes in cellular viability as determined by enzyme leakage

At present these approaches still require considerable further investigation to ascertain their predictive value and to work out the optimum procedures.

APPENDIX 15-1: PRIMARY IRRITATION*

Primary irritation of the skin is measured by a patch-test technique on the abraded and intact skin of the albino rabbit clipped free of hair. A minimum of six subjects is used per preparation tested. The method consists in introducing under a one-inch patch 0.5 ml (in case of liquids) or 0.5 g (in cases of solids and semisolids) of the test substance. It is also desirable in the case of solids to attempt solubilizing in an appropriate solvent (see above) and to apply the solution as for liquids. The animals are immobilized in an animal holder with patches secured in place by adhesive tape. The entire trunk of the animal is then wrapped with ruberized cloth for the entire 24-hour period of exposure. This latter procedure aids in maintaining the test patches in position, and, in addition, retards the evaporation of volatile substances. After the 24 hours of exposure the patches are removed and the resulting reactions are evaluated on the basis of scores in Table A-1.

Readings are made also after 72 hours, and the final score represents an average of 24- and 72-hour readings. An equal number of exposures are made on areas of skin which have been previously abraded. The abrasions are minor incisions through the stratum corneum, but not sufficiently deep to disturb the derma (that is, not sufficiently deep to produce bleeding).

The total erythema and edema scores are added in both the 24- and 72-hour readings, and the averages of the scores for intact and abraded skin are

*From Draize, 1959.

Table A-1 Evaluation of Skin Reactions

(1) Erythema and Eschar Formation	
No erythema	0
Very slight erythema (barely perceptible)	1
Well defined erythema	2
Moderate to severe erythema	3
Severe erythema (beet redness) to slight eschar formation (injuries in depth	4
Total possible erythema score	4
(2) Edema Formation	
No edema	0
Very slight edema (barely perceptible)	1
Slight edema (edges of area well defined by definite raising)	2
Moderate edema (raised approximately 1 mm)	3
Severe edema (raised more than 1 mm and extending beyond area of exposure)	4
Total possible edema score	4

combined; this combined average is referred to as the primary irritation index. It is useful for placing compounds in general groups with reference to irritant properties.

Compounds producing combined averages (primary irritation indexes) of 2 or less are only mildly irritating; whereas those with indexes from 2 to 5 are moderate irritants, and those with scores above 6 are considered severe irritants.

REFERENCES

Aoki, T., Parker, D., and Turk, J. L. (1969) Analysis of soluble antigens in guinea pig epidermis. I. An immunoelectrophoretic study with special reference to tissue-specific antigens and enzyme antigens. *Immunology* 16: 485–497.

Birmingham, D. L. (1977) Cutaneous absorption and systemic activity. In: *Cutaneous Toxicity*, pp. 53–62. Eds. V. A. Drill and P. Lazar. New York: Academic Press.

Brubaker, M. M. (1972) Urticarial reaction to ammonium persulfate. *Soc. Trans. Arch. Dermatol.* 106:413–414.

Carter, R. O., and Griffith, J. F. (1965) Experimental bases for the realistic assessment of safety of topical agents. *Toxicol. Appl. Pharmacol.* 7(Supp. 2):60–73.

Draize, J. H. (1959) Dermal toxicity. In: *Appraisal of the Safety of Chemicals in Foods, Drugs and Cosmetics*. Ed. Editorial Committee of the Association of Food and Drug Officials of the United States, P.O. Box 3425, York, Penn. 17402.

Epstein, J. H. (1977) Photocontact allergy in humans. In: *Dermatotoxicology and Pharmacology*, pp. 413–426. Eds. F. N. Marzulli and H. I. Maibach. Washington, D.C.: Hemisphere.

Griffith, J. F., and Buehler, E. V. (1977) Prediction of skin irritancy and sensitizing potential by testing with animals and man. In: *Cutaneous Toxicity*, pp. 155-174. Eds. V. A. Drill and P. Lazar. New York: Academic Press.

Harber, L. C., and Baer, R. L. (1972) Pathogenic mechanisms of drug-induced photosensitivity. *J. Invest. Dermatol.* 58:327-342.

Harber, L. S., and Shalita, A. R. (1977). Immunologically mediated contact photosensitivity in guinea pigs. In: *Dermatotoxicology and Pharmacology*, pp. 427-439. Eds. F. N. Marzulli and H. I. Maibach. Washington, D.C.: Hemisphere.

Hood, D. L. (1977) Practical and theoretical considerations in evaluating dermal safety. In: *Cutaneous Toxicity*, pp. 15-30. Eds. V. A. Drill and P. Lazar. New York: Academic Press.

Hunziker, N. (1977) Histology of contact dermatitis in humans and experimental animals. In: *Dermatotoxicology and Pharmacology*, pp. 373-411. Eds. F. N. Marzulli and H. I. Maibach. Washington, D.C.: Hemisphere.

IARC (1973) *Certain polycyclic aromatic hydrocarbons and heterocyclic compounds*. IARC Monographs on the Evaluation of Carcinogenic Risk of the Chemical to Man, Vol. 3. Lyon, France: International Agency for Research on Cancer.

IARC (1979) *Chemicals and industrial processes associated with cancer in humans*. IARC Monographs Supplement 1. Lyon, France: International Agency for Research on Cancer.

Jacobs, J. L. (1940) Immediate generalized skin reactions in hypersensitive guinea pigs. *Proc. Soc. Exp. Biol. Med.* 43:641-643.

Klecak, G. (1977) Identification of contact allergens: Predictive tests in animals. In: *Dermatotoxicology and Pharmacology*, pp. 305-339. Eds. F. N. Marzulli and H. I. Maibach. Washington, D.C.: Hemisphere.

Kligman, A. M., and Katz, A. G. (1968) Pathogenesis of acne vulgaris. I. Comedogenic properties of human sebum in external ear canal of the rabbit. *Arch. Dermatol.* 98:53-57.

Lahti, A., and Maibach, H. I. (1984) An animal model for nonimmunologic contact urticaria. *Toxicol. Appl. Pharmacol.* 76:219-224.

Magnusson, B., and Kligman, A. M. (1977) Usefulness of guinea pig tests for detection of contact sensitizers. In: *Dermatotoxicology and Pharmacology*, pp. 551-560. Eds. F. N. Marzulli and H. I. Maibach. Washington, D.C.: Hemisphere.

McCreesh, A. H., and Steinberg, M. L. (1977) Skin irritation testing in animals. In: *Dermatotoxicology and Pharmacology*, pp. 193-210. Eds. F. N. Marzulli and H. I. Maibach. Washington, D.C.: Hemisphere.

Middleton, M. C. (1981) New approaches to problems of dermatotoxicity. In: *Testing for Toxicity*. Ed. J. W. Gorrod. London: Taylor & Francis.

Montagna, W. (1965) The skin. *Sci. Am.* (Feb.):60.

Nixon, G. A., Tyson, C. A., and Werz, W. C. (1975) Interspecies comparisons of skin irritancy. *Toxicol. Appl. Pharmacol.* 31:481-490.

Odom, R. B., and Maibach, H. I. (1977) Contact urticaria: A different contact dermititis. In: *Dermatotoxicology and Pharmacology*, pp. 441-453. Eds. F. N. Marzulli and H. I. Maibach. Washington, D.C.: Hemisphere.

Pearson, R. S. B. (1966) Potato sensitivity: An occupational allergen in housewaves. *Acta Allerg.* 21:507-514.

Phillips, L., II, et al. (1972) A comparison of rabbit and human skin response to certain irritants. *Toxicol. Appl. Pharmacol.* 21:369–382.

Pocchiari, F. (1980) Accidental release of 2,3,7,8-tetrachlorodibenzo-*p*-dioxin (TCDD) at Seveso, Italy. *Ecotoxicol. Environ. Safety* 4:282.

Polak, L. (1977) Immunological aspects of contact sensitivity. In: *Dermatoxicology and Pharmacology*, pp. 225–288. Eds. F. N. Marzulli and H. I. Maibach. Washington, D.C.: Hemisphere.

Reeves, J. R. T., and Maibach, H. I. (1977) Drug and chemical induced hair loss. In: *Dermatotoxicology and Pharmacology*, pp. 487–500. Eds. F. N. Marzulli and H. I. Maibach. Washington, D.C.: Hemisphere.

Reller, H. H., and Luedders, W. L. (1977) Pharmacologic and toxicologic effects of topically applied agents on the eccrine sweat glands. In: *Dermatotoxicology and Pharmacology*, pp. 1–54. Eds. F. N. Marzulli and H. I. Maibach. Washington, D.C.: Hemisphere.

Roudabush, R. L., et al. (1965) Comparative acute effects of some chemicals on the skin of rabbits and guinea pigs. *Toxicol. Appl. Pharmacol.* 7:559–565.

Shelley, W. B., and P. N. Horvath (1950) Experimental miliaria in man. II. Production of sweat retention anhidrosis and miliaria crystallina by various kinds of injury. *J. Invest. Dermatol.* 1:9–20.

Weil, C. S., and Scala, R. A. (1973) Study of intra- and interlaboratory variability in the results of rabbit eye and skin irritation tests. *Toxicol. Appl. Pharmacol.* 19:276–360.

WHO (1976) *Polychlorinated Biphenyls and Terphenyls*. Environmental Health Criteria 2. Geneva: World Health Organization.

Chapter 16

Toxicology of the Eye

GENERAL CONSIDERATIONS

Although the eyes are relatively small, they are important to one's well-being and they are complex in structure.

The eye is a spherical body that is covered mainly by three coats of tissues: the sclera, choroid, and retina. These coats mainly consist of, respectively, fibrous tissues, pigments and blood vessels, and nerve fibers, cells, and special receptors. They are nontransparent. However, light is admitted through the front of the eye, where the three coats are replaced by a number of tissues, notably the cornea and the lens (Fig. 16-1a).

The cornea is a continuum of the sclera. It consists of a relatively thick stroma and is covered, in front, by an epithelium, consisting of several layers of cells and Bowman's membranes, and, behind, by Descemet's membrane and an endothelium. The cornea and the front portion of the sclera as well as the inside of the eyelids are covered by a thin layer of conjunctiva.

The lens consists of transparent fibers enclosed in the lens capsule. It is suspended by the ciliary zonule to the ciliary body and its curvature is adjustable by the contraction and relaxation of the ciliary muscle.

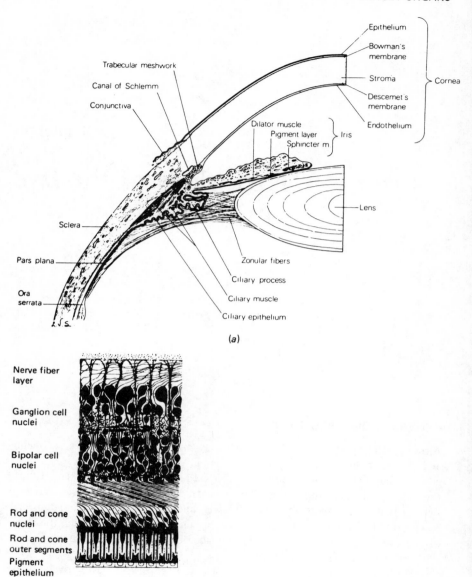

Figure 16-1 (a) Cross section of the anterior chamber angle and surrounding structures. (Reproduced, with permission, from Vaughan, D., Asbury, T. *General Ophthalmology*, 10th ed. Copyright © 1983 by Lange Medical Publications, Los Altos, Calif.) (b) Cross section of the retina. (Reproduced, with permission of the author, from Polyak, S. *The Retina*. Copyright © 1940 by University of Chicago Press, Chicago, Ill.)

The space between the lens and the cornea is filled with the aqueous humor. Also in this space and immediately in front of the lens is the iris. It is rich in blood vessels and heavily pigmented. The iris has a central opening, the pupil. Filling the space between the lens and retina is the vitreous humor.

The retina is the ocular structure that responds to light stimuli. It consists of several layers (Fig. 16-1b). The outermost is a pigmented epithelium. Next to it are the retinal rods and cones, which are the light-responsive neural structures. They are connected via the bipolar cells to the ganglion cells. The axons from the latter cells converge and exit from the eye at the optic papilla.

Because of their diverse physiologic nature and spatial relations, these various ocular structures may exhibit a variety of effects as a result of exposure to toxicants.

SITE AND TYPE OF TOXIC EFFECTS

Cornea

The cornea is a delicate structure and is subject to toxic effects of chemicals, mainly from external exposure. Chemicals that affect the cornea include acids and alkalies, detergents, organic solvents, and smog. Acids and alkalies can readily damage the cornea. The extent of damage ranges from minor, superficial destruction of the tissue, which heals completely, to opacity of the cornea or even perforation. Acid burns are related to the low pH as well as the affinity of the anion for the corneal tissue. The effects of alkalies usually have slower onset than those caused by acids and are essentially pH-dependent. However, ammonium ion, which is present in many household products, penetrates the cornea more readily and can thereby affect the iris (Potts and Gonasun, 1980).

Detergents are useful household and industrial products. In general, the nonionic detergents are less damaging than the ionic agents, and the cationics are more damaging than the anionics (Draize and Kelley, 1952). Organic solvents, such as acetone, hexane, and toluene, may enter the eye as a result of industrial or laboratory accidents. These substances can dissolve fat and damage the corneal epithelial cells.

Smog is a mixture of industrial smoke and fog. However, it now refers more often to the photochemical reaction products of automobile exhaust. These products accumulate under certain meteorologic conditions. They affect mainly the respiratory tract, but even at low concentrations they irritate the corneal sensory nerve endings and cause reflex lacrimation.

Other chemicals can affect the cornea following *systemic administration*. These include quinacrine, chloroquine, and chlorpromazine. Potts and Gonasun (1980) reviewed the corneal effects of these drugs and other chemicals. These chemicals affect the cornea likely via tears and/or after passing through the blood-aqueous barrier. However, they affect humans only rarely and only after large doses.

Iris, Aqueous Humor, and Ciliary Body

Because of its proximity to the cornea, the *iris* is susceptible to physical trauma and chemical irritation. The effects of such irritation consists of leakage of serum proteins and fibrin from the blood vessels as well as leukocytes. These may be followed by fibroblast metaplasia. Severe damages to the iris cause liberation of melanin granules from the posterior epithelium of the iris.

The iris is innervated by sympathetic nerves (for the dilator muscles) and parasympathetic nerves (for the constrictor muscles). Therefore, the pupil can be dilated by chemicals that are sympathomimetic or parasympatholytic, and it can be constricted by parasympathomimetic and sympatholytic chemicals. Furthermore the size of the pupil can be altered via the central nervous system by chemicals such as morphine and general anesthetics.

The *aqueous humor* is secreted by the epithelium of the ciliary body into the posterior chamber. It flows through the pupil into the anterior chamber and drains through the canal of Schlemm at the angle of the anterior chamber. Inflammatory changes of the iris can block the drainage of the fluid through the canal of Schlemm and raise the intraocular pressure, thereby inducing glaucoma. Atropine and other mydriatics may also precipitate glaucoma by blocking the drainage.

In the *ciliary body* is the ciliary muscle, the contraction of which allows relaxation of the ciliary zonule, which in turn allows the lens capsule to assume a more spherical form. This muscle is parasympathetically innervated; therefore, cholinesterase inhibitors and parasympatholytic agents such as atropine can cause the lens to be fixed in different state of accommodation.

Lens

A number of chemicals are known to alter the lenticular transparency, resulting in the formation of cataract. Examples are 2,4-dinitrophenol, corticosteroids, busulfan, triparanol, and thallium. Their cataractogenic property has been noted in humans as well as animals, such as the rabbit, rat, and young fowl. The effects generally follow systemic exposure, but with certain chemicals (e.g., corticosteroids, anticholinesterases), they may occur after topical application (Becker, 1964; Woods et al., 1967; Axelsson, 1968).

Diabetic patients are more likely to have cataracts, which can also be produced in rats and rabbits rendered diabetic with alloxan or streptozotocin (Heywood, 1982).

In addition, rats fed large amounts of galactose develop cataract (Sippel, 1966). This condition may be comparable to the cataract observed in infants with galactosemia. Such galactosemia results from a metabolic inability, inherited as an autosomal recessive trait, to convert galactose to glucose because of absence of the enzyme galactose-1-phosphate uridylyl transference (Kinosita, 1965).

On the other hand, deficiencies of certain nutrients may also induce cataract. These nutrients include tryptophan, proteins, vitamin E, riboflavin, and folic acid (Gehring, 1971).

The mechanism underlying the formation of cataract is not fully understood. It is likely that it varies with the nature of the toxicant. For example, corticosteroid cataract may be mediated through an inhibition of protein synthesis in the lens (Ono, 1972). Busulfan may act through an interference of mitosis of the lenticular epithelial cells (Grimes and von Sallmann, 1966). Triparanol may interfere with the Na^+ pump, resulting in an increase of Na^+ and water in the lens (Harris and Gruber, 1972).

An extensive review of cataractogenic chemicals has been prepared by Gehring (1971). These chemicals are listed in Appendix 16-1.

Apart from cataractogenic effects, transient lens opacity may be induced by certain chemicals. For example, these have been noted in young beagle dogs following administration of some tranquilizers, some diuretics, and diisophenol. In addition, the transparency and refraction of the lens may also be altered by dimethyl sulfoxide and p-chlorophenylalanine (Heywood, 1982).

Retina

Certain polycyclic compounds, such as chloroquine, hydroxychloroquine, and thioridazine, can induce retinopathy in humans and animals. They affect the visual acuity, dark adaptation, and retinal pigment pattern. Hyperoxia and iodate also may induce retinal changes. Meier-Ruge (1972) reviewed the literature on various retinopathic chemicals.

Different mechanisms are involved in these retinal effects. Inhibition of protein metabolism in the pigment epithelium has been suggested as the primary toxic effect of chloroquine and hydroxychloroquine, which have strong affinity for melanin (Meier-Ruge, 1972). Increased oxygen supply to the retina induces vasoconstriction, which is associated with a decrease in the supply of nutrients. The latter effect is probably responsible for the hyperoxia-induced retinal changes (Nichols and Lambertson, 1969). Iodate apparently affects the pigment epithelium, the derangement of which results in degeneration of the rod layer (Graymore and Tansley, 1959). A recent review of the various modes of action has been provided by Heywood (1982). These include the early formation of membranous cytoplasmic bodies (myeloid bodies), degenerative changes in the cell body of the rods and cones, derangement of the intracytoplasmic rods, and the appearing of vacuoles around these rods in the tapetum (Heywood, 1982).

Other retinal effects include hemorrhage from rupture of blood vessels or disturbance of blood clotting mechanism and exudates, which may cause partial detachment of retina (Heywood, 1982).

Optic Nerve

As noted in Chapter 1, the retina contains, among other structures, the ganglion cells the axons of which form the optic nerve. Toxicants can affect either the ganglion cells or the optic nerve. Damage to one of them results in the degeneration of the other.

Some toxicants affect mainly the central vision. The most notable example is methanol. Others include carbon disulfide, disulfuram, ethambutol, and thallium. On the other hand, quinine, chloroquine, pentavalent arsenic, and carbon monoxide cause constriction of visual fields by damaging the structures responsible for peripheral vision. Interestingly, nitrobenzol affects both the central and peripheral vision (Harrington, 1976).

These toxicants can also be classified according to their effects on other peripheral nerves. For example, quinine, ethambutol, and methanol generally do not affect other peripheral nerves, while carbon disulfide, disulfuram, and thallium cause both optic and peripheral neuropathies. It is worthy of note that certain organic solvents can induce peripheral neuropathy but spare the visual system. These include tri-o-cresyl phosphate, acrylamide, n-hexane, and methyl n-butyl ketone (Grant, 1980).

In general, the mode of action is not well understood; however, quinine appears to act through an inhibition DNA, which in turn inhibits RNA transcription and protein synthesis. Pentavalent arsenic appears to act on the ganglion cell neurons (Potts and Gonasun, 1980).

TESTING PROCEDURES

Effects on the eye can be examined after topical application of the toxicants. In certain cases, systemic administration can also result in ocular alterations. Several types of examinations are available.

Albino rabbits are commonly used to determine the ocular irritancy of ophthalmic medications and other chemicals that might come in contact with the eye. Dogs and nonhuman primates (rhesus monkeys) have also been used (Beckley, 1964). For effects on the lens, retina, and optical nerve, many species of animals are used, e.g., rat, rabbit, cat, dog, monkey, and pig.

Gross Examination

The test described by Draize and Kelley (1952) has been a standard procedure for testing ocular irritancy. It specifies the use of nine rabbits. Into one eye of each rabbit is instilled 0.1 ml of the test material. In three of the nine rabbits, the test material is washed with 20 ml of lukewarm water 2 seconds after the instillation, and in three others, the washing is done with a 4-second delay. In the three remaining rabbits, the material is left in the eye. The ocular reactions are read with the unaided eye or with the aid of a hand slip lamp at 24, 48, and

72 hours and at 4 and 7 days after treatment. The reactions of the conjunctiva (redness, chemosis, and discharge), cornea (the degree and extent of opacity), and iris (congestion, swelling, and circumcorneal injection) are scored according to a specified scale. A series of colored pictures, originally provided by the U.S. Food and Drug Administration in 1965, as a guide for grading eye irritation were reproduced in McDonald and Shadduck, 1977.

Several modified versions of the Draize and Kelley test have been proposed. Griffith et al. (1980) reported on their results of assessing eye irritancy of a large number of substances. The irritancy ranged from nil to corrosive. The authors recommend that the following points be taken into account in conducting eye irritation tests:

1 A 0.01-ml dose, or its weight equivalent for solids and powders, be applied directly to the central corneal surface of at least six eyes without subsequent rinsing or manipulation of the eyelids

2 Evaluation of the irritancy be based on the median duration for the eyes to return to normal, instead of using a scoring system based on the type and extent of the effects.

The latest U.S. federal agency regulation (CPSC, 1983) requires the use of six albino rabbits for each test substance. For test liquids, 0.1 ml is used, and for solids and pastes, 100 mg. The test material is instilled into one eye of each rabbit without washing. Ocular examinations are done after 24, 48, and 72 hours. A rabbit is considered as having positive reaction if the eye shows, on any examination, ulceration or opacity of the cornea, inflammation of the iris, or swelling of the conjunctiva with partial eversion of the eyelids.

Another variation of the Draize procedure calls for the use of three rabbits whose eyes are examined at 1, 24, 48, and 72 hours. If there are signs of irritation, six additional rabbits are tested, half of which are washed four seconds after the instillation of the test substance, and the other half washed 30 seconds after the instillation. This is done continuously for five minutes (OECD, 1981).

Instrumental Examinations

Ophthalmoscopy The ophthalmoscope is required in assessing effects of toxicants on various parts of the retina. The examination is generally intended to discover the existence of edema, hyperemia or pallor, atrophy of the optic disk, pigmentation, or the state of the blood vessels. Changes in the vitreous humor, lens, aqueous humor, iris, and cornea can also be discovered.

Visual Perimetry Effect on the visual field can be readily determined in humans, but not in laboratory animals, except the nonhuman primates. Merigan (1979) described a procedure using macaque monkeys to demonstrate the loss of peripheral vision resulting from exposure to methyl mercury.

Other Procedures Visual acuity and color vision are sensitive and useful indicators of effects on the visual system in humans. Procedures involving instrumentation, e.g., electro-oculography, and visual-evoked responses are also useful and can be incorporated in animal experimentation (Grant, 1980). The usefulness and limitations of new procedures, including neurotoxic, neuro-chemical, and behavioral approaches for the study of toxic effects on the visual cortical receptive field, have been reviewed by Sinkman et al. (1982).

Histologic and Biochemical Examinations

Light microscopy can usually pinpoint the site of action of toxicants. Electron microscopy can demonstrate ultrastructural changes, and biochemical studies can reveal the mechanism of toxic effects. For example, chloroquine has been observed with light microscopy to cause a thickening of the pigment epithelium, followed by migration of the pigment to the outer nuclear layer, and finally total atrophy of the photoreceptors (Meier-Ruge, 1968). Electron microscopy showed mitochondrial swelling and disorganization of the endoplasmic reticulum in the photoreceptor inner segment (Solze and McConnell, 1970). Biochemical studies revealed inhibition of many enzymatic reactions, especially those related to protein metabolism of the pigment epithelium.

EVALUATION

Eye irritation tests are widely used to assess the ocular irritancy of chemicals. In general, the albino rabbit is the animal of choice. Some intralaboratory and interlaboratory variations in the scores were noted in two collaborative studies (Weil and Scala, 1971; Marzulli and Ruggles, 1973). Nevertheless, periodic collaborative studies tend to improve the reliability of the scores. The various modifications made on the Draize test also tend to reduce the variability of the results.

Despite the variability of the results, the tests in rabbits have proved useful in predicting eye irritation in humans. It is worth noting that the test in rabbits in some instances showed greater irritancy than that encountered in human use (McDonald and Shadduck, 1977).

A large number of animal experimentations and clinical studies indicate that there is a fair correlation between humans and animals in their reactions to toxicants with respect to cataract formation and retinopathy (Grant, 1980; Potts and Gonasun, 1980).

APPENDIX 16-1: CATARACTOGENIC CHEMICALS

Sugars (glucose, galactose, xylose)	Anticholinesterases
Streptozotocin	Chlorpromazine
Corticosteroids	Triparanol

Naphthalene
Tyrosine
2,4-Dinitrophenol (DNP) and related
    compounds
Alkylating agents
Mimosine (leucenol)
Methoxsalen
Methionine sulphoximine
Polyriboinosinic acid polyribocytidylic
    acid
Quietidine (1,4-bis(phenylisopropyl)-
    piperazine 2 HCl
N-Phenyl-β-hydrazinopropionitriles
    and related compounds
4[3(7-Chloro-5,11-dihydrodibenz-
    [b,e] [1,4]-oxazepin-5-YL)propyl]-
    1-piperazineethanol dichloride

Dimethyl sulfoxide (DMSO)
2,4,6-Trinitrotoluene (TNT)
Sympathomimetic drugs and
    morphine-like drugs
2,6-Dichloro-4-nitroaniline
Iodoacetic acid
Mephenytoin
Diquat
Oral contraceptives
Sulfaethoxypyridazine
Thallium
Paradichlorobenzene
Heptachlor
Desferal
Thioacetamide

REFERENCES

Axelsson, U. (1968) Glaucoma, miotic therapy and cataract. III. Visual loss due to lens changes in glaucoma eyes treated with paraoxon (Mintacol), echothiophate or pilocarpine. *Acta Ophthalmol.* 46:831.

Becker, B. (1964) Cataract and topical corticosteroids. *Am. J. Ophthalmol.* 58: 872–873.

Beckley, J. H. (1964) Comparative eye testing: Man vs. animal. *Toxicol. Appl. Pharmacol.* 7:93–101.

CPSC (1983) Consumer Product Safety Commission. Test for eye irritants. Code of Federal Regulations, Title 16. Federal Hazardous Substances Act Regulation, Part 1500.42.

Draize, J. H., and Kelley, E. A. (1952) Toxicity to eye mucosa of certain cosmetic preparations containing surface-active agents. *Proc. Sci. Sect. Toilet Goods Assoc.* 17:1–4.

Gehring, P. J. (1971) The cataractogenic activity of chemical agents. *CRC Crit. Rev. Toxicol.* 1:93–118.

Grant, W. M. (1980) The peripheral visual system as a target. In: *Experimental and Clinical Neurotoxicology*. Eds. B. S. Spencer and H. H. Schaumburg. Baltimore: Williams & Wilkins.

Graymore, C. N., and Tansley, K. C. (1959) Iodoacetate poisoning of the rat retina. *Br. J. Ophthalmol.* 43:177–185.

Griffith, J. F., et al. (1980) Dose-response studies with chemical irritants in the albino rabbit eye as a basis for selecting optimum testing conditions for predicting hazard to the human eye. *Toxicol. Appl. Pharmacol.* 55:501–513.

Grimes, P., and Von Sallmann, L. (1966) Interference with cell proliferation and induction of polyploidy in rat lens epithelium during prolonged Myleran treatment. *Exp. Cell Res.* 62:265–273.

Harrington, D. O. (1976) *The Visual Fields.* St. Louis: Mosby.

Harris, J. E., and Gruber, L. (1972) Reversal of triparanol-induced cataracts in the rat. II. Exchange of ^{22}Na, ^{42}K, ^{86}Rb in cataractous and clearing lenses. *Invest. Ophthalmol. Vis. Sci.* 11:608–616.

Heywood, R. (1982) Histopathological and laboratory assessment of visual dysfunction. *Environ. Health Perspect.* 44:35–45.

Kinosita, J. H. (1965) Cataracts in galactosemia. *Invest. Ophthalmol. Vis. Sci.* 4:786–799.

Marzulli, F. N., and Ruggles, D. I. (1973) Rabbit eye irritation test: Collaborative study. *J. Am. Assoc. Anal. Chem.* 56:905–914.

McDonald, T. O., and Shadduck, J. A. (1977) Eye irritation. In: *Dermatotoxicology and Pharmacology.* Eds. F. N. Marzulli and H. I. Maibach. Washington, D.C.: Hemisphere.

Meier-Ruge, M. (1968) The pathophysiological morphology of the pigment epithelium and its importance for retinal structure and function. *Med. Prob. Ophthalmol.* 8:32–48.

Meier-Ruge, W. (1972) Drug-induced retinopathy. *CRC Crit. Rev. Toxicol.* 1:325–360.

Merigan, W. H. (1979) Effects of toxicants on visual systems. *Neurobehav. Toxicol.* 1(Suppl. 1):15–22.

Nichols, C. W., and Lambertson, C. J. (1969) Effects of high oxygen pressures on the eye. *N. Engl. J. Med.* 281:25–30.

OECD (1981) *OECD Guidelines for Testing of Chemicals.* Paris: Organization for Economic Cooperation and Development.

Ono, S. (1972) Presence of corticol-binding protein in the lens. *Ophthalmic Res.* 3:233–240.

Potts, A. M., and Gonasun, L. M. (1980) Toxic responses of the eye. In: *Casarett and Doull's Toxicology.* Eds. J. Doull, C. D. Klaassen, and M. O. Amdur. New York: Macmillan.

Sinkman, P. G., Isley, M. R., and Rogers, D. C. (1982) Newer laboratory approaches for assessing visual dysfunction. *Environ. Health Perspect.* 44:55–62.

Sippel, T. O. (1966) Changes in water, protein and glutathione contents of the lens in the course of galactose cataract development in rats. *Invest. Ophthalmol. Vis. Sci.* 5:568–575.

Solze, D. A., and McConnell, D. G. (1970) Ultrastructural changes in the rat photoreceptor inner segment during experimental chloroquine retinopathy. *Ophthal. Res.* 1:140–148.

Weil, C. S., and Scala, R. A. (1971) Study of intra- and interlaboratory variability in the results of the rabbit eye and skin irritation test. *Toxicol. Appl. Pharmacol.* 19:276–360.

Woods, D. C., Contaxis, I., Sweet, D., Smith, J. C., II, and Van Dolah, J. (1967) Response of rabbits to corticosteroids. I. Influence on growth, intraocular pressure and lens transparency. *Am. J. Ophthalmol.* 63:841–849.

ADDITIONAL READINGS

Bernstein, H. N., Mills, D. W., and Becker, B. (1963) Steroid-induced elevation of intraocular pressure. *Arch. Ophthalmol.* 70:15–18.

Grant, W. M. (1974) *Toxicology of the Eye*, 2d ed. Springfield, Ill.: Charles C Thomas.

Chapter 17

Toxicology
of the Nervous
System

INTRODUCTION

As a vital part of the body, the nervous system is shielded by a unique protective mechanism, namely, the blood-brain and blood-nerve barriers. Nonetheless, it is susceptible to a variety of toxicants. For example, methyl mercury affects mainly the nervous system, although its concentration in the brain is comparable to that in most other tissues, and in fact it is much lower than that in the liver and kidneys.

The greater susceptibility may be attributed partly to the fact that neurons have a high metabolic rate, with little capacity for anaerobic metabolism. Furthermore, being electrically excitable, neurons tend to lose cell membrane integrity more readily. The great length of the axons is another reason why the nervous system is especially susceptible to toxic effects, since the cell body must supply its axon structurally and metabolically.

To facilitate the description of the various types of toxic effects and the procedures for their testing, the various parts of the nervous system are presented.

Central and Peripheral Nervous Systems

The system consists of two major parts: the central nervous system (CNS) and the peripheral nervous system (PNS). The former is made up of the brain and the spinal cord and the latter includes the cranial and spinal nerves, which are either motor or sensory. The neurons of the sensory spinal nerves are located in the ganglia in the dorsal roots. In addition, the PNS also includes the sympathetic nerve system, which arises from neurons in the thoracic and lumbar region of the spinal cord, and the parasympathetic system, which stems from nerve fibers leaving the CNS via the cranial nerves and the sacral spinal roots.

Cells and Appendages

The principal cells in the nervous system are neurons along with their axons. These structures are responsible for the conduction of nerve impulses. The main supporting structure consists of various types of glial cells. Apart from a lack of conductivity, the glial cells differ from neurons in that the former, as most other types of cells, do reproduce whereas the latter do not.

In the CNS the glial cells include astrocytes, oligodendrocytes (oligodendroglia), and microglia. Astrocytes help maintain a proper microenvironment around the neurons and support the blood-brain barrier. Oligodendroglia surround the axons in the CNS with a lipid-rich material, the myelin sheath, which provides electrical insulation. Microglia are basically macrophages that are located in the CNS. In the PNS the Schwann cells wrap around the axons to provide the myelin sheath, which is interrupted by the nodes of Ranvier.

Neurons are connected, via their axons, to other neurons at their dendrites or to the receptors in the glands or muscles. At nerve terminals, on excitation by an action potential, chemical neurotransmitters are released. The most common transmitters are acetylcholine and norepinephrine. However, there are many others. For example, a list of 25 chemicals that may function as central neurotransmitter and neuromodulators has been compiled by Blatteis (1981).

Blood-Brain and Blood-Nerve Barriers

These barriers protect the nervous system from certain neurotoxins. Difference in neurotoxicity sometimes can be explained on the basis of these barriers.

Blood-Brain Barrier (BBB) The endothelium is impermeable to substances of medium molecular weight, such as horseradish peroxidase (mol. wt.: 40,000; diameter: 5-6 nm), because the adjacent cells are tightly joined. Further, these cells have few micropinocytotic vesicles, which in capillaries of other tissues serve as an important transport mechanism across endothelial cells. However, highly lipid-soluble substances and the nonionized fraction of a chemical are more permeable across the BBB. It is, therefore, similar to intact cell membranes in permeability.

The BBB is absent where the cells produce hormones or act as hormonal or chemoreceptors. Glutamate and a number of related compounds, such as aspartate, have been shown to affect areas in the brain not protected by the BBB, e.g., the arcuate nucleus of the hypothalamus and the area postrema in various laboratory animals. These effects, while not observed in humans, are of interest because they may be used as tools in the study of such clinical conditions as Huntington's disease, drug-induced parkinsonism, tardive dyskinesia, and sulfur amino acidopathies.

The BBB is effective in excluding many neurotoxins, such as diphtheria, staphylococcus, and tetanus toxins. This is also true with doxorubicin, which affects the dorsal root ganglia but not the CNS. Mercury chloride has a small molecule but is hydrophilic and mainly in ionic forms. Its concentration in the brain is minimal and so are its CNS effects. On the other hand, methyl mercury is lipophilic and thus readily crosses the BBB, thereby damaging the brain.

Blood-Nerve Barrier (BNB) Peripheral nerves are covered by two connective tissue sheaths, the perineurium and epineurium, and interlaced with the endoneurium. The BNB is provided by the blood vessels in the endoneurium and supplemented by the lamellated cells of the perineural sheath. It is not as effective as the BBB; therefore, the dorsal root glanglia are generally more susceptible than the neurons in the CNS to neurotoxins (Jacobs, 1980).

CATEGORIES OF NEUROTOXIC EFFECTS

The effects may be classified according to the site of action. These include the cell body and other parts of the neurons, especially the axons, the glial cells, and the vascular system. A toxicant may affect one or more sites. The following is a brief description of various neurotoxic effects, along with the putative mode of action, grouped according to the sites of action. Figure 17-1 shows the main categories of neurotoxic effects.

Neuronopathy

Neurons, being dependent mainly on glucose as an energy source, are susceptible to anoxic and hypoglycemic conditions. A number of chemicals are well known for their anoxigenic effects in the brain (Norton, 1980a). Barbiturates induce anoxia in the brain, especially in certain areas of the cerebral cortex, hippocampus, and cerebellum. Permanent CNS damage even after barbiturate coma, however, is rare. On the other hand, prolonged exposure to carbon monoxide may induce permanent effects in the brain, arising from the development of a diffuse sclerosis of the white matter (leukoencephalopathy). Cyanide and azide inhibit cytochrome oxidase, thereby producing cytotoxic anoxia.

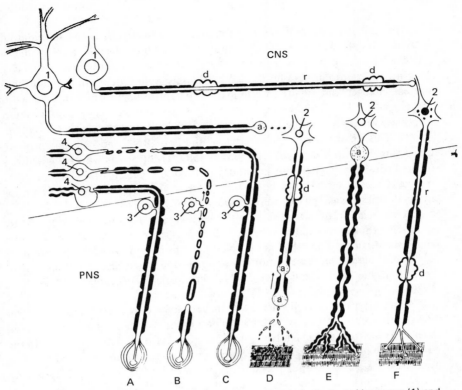

Figure 17-1 Cellular target sites of some neurotoxic chemicals illustrated by upper (1) and lower (2) motor neurons, dorsal root ganglion cells (3), and second order sensory neurons (4) in the gracile nucleus of the medulla oblongata. The central nervous system (CNS) is represented above the sloping horizontal line, the peripheral nervous system (PNS) below. The peripheral receptors on fibers a–c are pacinian corpuscles. Fibers d–f innervate extrafusal muscle fibers. (A) Neuronopathy: The excitotoxin alanosine acts as a false transmitter at neuron 4 causing maintained depolarization leading to cellular damage (B) Neuronopathy: Doxorubicin irreversibly damages neuron 3 resulting a rapid anterograde (arrows) pattern of total axonal breakdown and myelin loss. (C) Central distal axonopathy: Clioquinol induced retrograde degeneration of the central axonal process of the dorsal root ganglion cell (3) but leaves the cell and peripheral process intact. (D) Central-peripheral distal axonopathy: 2,5-Hexanedione causes retrograde axonal degeneration (a) to develop slowly in long and large central and peripheral axons. Muscle atrophy will occur unless axons regenerate and sprouts reinnervate the muscle. The anterior horn cell (2) is left intact, and eventually (after months to years) a secondary demyelination in the ventral root ensues (d). (E) IDPN causes a giant axonal swelling (a) to develop in the intraspinal portion of the axon; the distal axon attenuates but does not degenerate. (F) Myelinopathy: AETT causes myelin bubbling (d) focally along the axon of large diameter central (1) and peripheral (2) axons. Axonal denudation is followed by remyelination: this is occurring in the ventral roots (r) and medulla oblongata when demyelination (d) is in progress in the peripheral nerve and elsewhere. A similar process would occur in a primary disease of the myelinating cell except that remyelination might not occur during intoxication. (From Spencer, P. S., and Schaumberg, H. H. Eds. *Experimental and Clinical Neurotoxicology*. Baltimore: William & Wilkins. Copyright © 1980, with permission.)

The cell body of neurons may be affected directly by toxicants. Methyl mercury first causes focal loss of ribosomes and then disintegration and disappearance of the Nissl substances. These effects lead to an imparied capacity to synthesize protein (Cavanagh, 1977). This is followed by nuclear and perinuclear changes and finally by the loss of the entire neuron including its axon (Jacobs et al., 1975; 1977). Doxorubicin (Adriamycin) affects neurons by intercalating with DNA, leading to a breakdown of the helical structures (Cho et al., 1980). This derangement inhibits the synthesis of RNA and neuronal protein. Since this drug does not cross the blood-brain barrier, it can affect the neurons in the dorsal root glangia but not those in the CNS. On the other hand, methyl mercury does penetrate the blood-brain barrier and thus damages the neurons in the dorsal root glanglia as well as those in the CNS.

Accumulation of neurofibrils in the perikarya and axons may be caused by vincristine (Schoental and Cavanagh, 1977). It disrupts the axonal neurotubules and neurofilaments and blocks axoplasmic transport of these ultrastructures. Aluminum also induces neurofibrillar degeneration in cat and rabbit and might be responsible for certain cases of Alzheimer's disease (Crapper and DeBoni, 1980).

Glutamate and related chemicals, in very large doses, are known to affect areas of the CNS devoid of BBB (see Blood-Brain Barrier section) and are considered as having neuroexcitatory and neurotoxic effects. The dendrites are the primary site of action. The perikarya are then affected, but the axons are spared. Kainic acid is derived from a particular seaweed and it has been used in ascariasis; it is similar to glutamate but much more potent (Olney, 1980).

Axonopathy

Some axons are very long (up to 1 meter), and the elements in the axons, such as neurofibrils, are synthesized not locally but in the cell body and are transported along the axon. The axon may therefore be attacked either directly by toxicants or indirectly through damages to the cell body.

Lesions may occur either in the proximal or in the distal sections of axons.

Proximal Axonopathy β,β-Iminodiproprionitrile (IDPN) produces typical lesions of this type. It has, therefore, been used as a model to study motor neuron diseases such as amyotrophic lateral sclerosis. The primary effect of IDPN is the impairment of slow axonal transport of neurofilaments while their synthesis is continued in the cell body. The accumulation of neurofilaments in the proximal axon causes it to enlarge and the distal axon to atrophy. The enlarged proximal axon in turn elicits local proliferation of the subpial astrocytic processes and extension of the processes filled with glial filaments along the proximal ventral root. The proximal swelling also stimulates splitting of myelin at the intraperiod line, formation of intramyelinic vacuoles, and ultimate demyelination. The Schwann cells in the demyelinated segment divide and remyelinate, and the repeated demyelination and remyelination give rise to "onion-bulb" formation (Griffin and Price, 1980).

Distal Axonopathy Axons contain three types of neurofibrillary structures, namely, neurotubules, neurofilaments, and microfilaments. In addition, they contain mitochondria and smooth endoplasmic reticulum. These structures are especially susceptible to a variety of neurotoxicants. For example, thallium induces mitochondrial swelling and degeneration, and certain organophosphates and organic solvents cause derangement of the neurofibrillary structures, resulting in distal axonopathy.

An important type of distal axonopathy is produced by certain organophosphorous compounds such as TOCP (tri-*o*-cresyl phosphate) and leptophos. These compounds, besides inhibiting cholinesterase, cause *delayed neuropathy*, which manifests mainly as paralysis of muscles. It affects especially long and large nerve fibers, hence the hindlimbs are paralyzed before the forelimbs. Although a number of other animals may also be affected, especially after repeated exposures, this toxicity can be readily reproduced in hens, usually with a delay of 8–10 days after exposure. Because of the severity of delayed neurotoxicity, new organophosphorous chemicals are routinely tested for this potential hazard. OECD (1984) has published guidelines for such tests both after a single dose and after repeated administrations, using domestic hens. The condition is unrelated to cholinesterase inhibition because such potent inhibitors as malathion, parathion, and carbaryl do not possess this toxic property. It is apparently associated with phosphorylation of the enzyme neurotoxic esterase. Additional details and references are provided by Davis and Richardson (1980).

A different type of distal axonopathy is known to be caused by hexacarbons such as *n*-hexane and methyl *n*-butyl ketone. These solvents have caused toxic polyneuropathy among industrial workers, as has acrylamide. Both cause marked neurofilament proliferation in axons. However, giant axonal swellings are common with hexacarbons but rare with acrylamide. Furthermore, sensory nerves are involved early with acrylamide but late with hexacarbons, which affect certain motor nerves first. The lesions induced by acrylamide, hexacarbons, and organophosphates are all distal but preterminal (Asbury and Brown, 1980).

Distal axonopathy has been hypothesized as resulting from impairment of glycolytic enzyme activities in the axon (Spencer et al., 1979). These enzymes are responsible for the transport of neurofilaments, which are synthesized in the perikaryon and transported along the axon. Impairment of the activities of these enzymes would thus first affect the distal portion of the axon as well as the large, long nerve fibers, which have a great energy demand on the perikarya.

A second hypothesis postulates that the neurofilaments are directly affected by toxicants such as hexacarbons and acrylamide (Savolainen, 1977; Politis et al., 1980). Neurofilaments exposed to the toxicant for the longest period, namely, those located distally in long fibers, would be affected first.

Blockade of Impulse Conduction A number of toxicants act mainly on nerve membranes. These membranes normally maintain a negative resting potential. When stimulated, an action potential is generated. The resting and action potentials result from differences in the Na^+ and K^+ concentrations across the membrane, and their concentrations are maintained by the Na^+ and K^+ pumps. Tetrodotoxin, the toxic principle of puffer fish, has been shown to block the action potential by blocking the Na^+ pump. Saxitoxin, the toxic principle produced by the dinoflagellate *Gonyaulax* and taken up by the clam *Saxidomas giganteus*, also acts by blocking the sodium pump. Consumption of improperly cleaned puffer fish or contaminated clam can cause death by respiratory failure. The binding with saxitoxin, however, is more readily reversible. These toxins have been useful tools in investigating the mode of action of neurotoxins (Narahashi, 1980).

Blockade of Synaptic Transmission Botulinus toxin, the most potent biologic toxin, is produced by *Clostridium botulinum*. It causes paralysis of muscles by impairing the release of the neurotransmitter acetylcholine from motor nerve endings. Black widow spider venom, on the other hand, causes a massive release of acetylcholine and results in cramps and paralysis.

A number of toxicants affect the neurotransmission in the CNS. For example, tetanoplasmin, from the microbe *Clostridium tetani*, causes tetanus. It disinhibits the motoneurons in the spinal cord by binding to the receptors on the neurons. The molecular weight of this proteinaceous dimer is about 150,000, therefore too large to cross the blood-brain barrier. However, it reaches the CNS by retrograde axonal transport (Schield et al., 1977). This retrograde transport normally serves in recycling materials originally transported from the cell body to the nerve ending.

Other toxicants affecting neurotransmission include boron hydrides (decrease norepinephrine and serotonin), carbon disulfide (decreases norepinephrine and increases dopamine), chlorodimeform (increases serotonin and norepinephrine) DDT and dieldrin (decrease acetylcholine and norepinephrine), and manganese (decreases serotonin, norepinephrine, and dopamine). Some details on these effects have been given by Damstra and Bondy (1980).

Glial Cells and Myelin

Myelinating Cells Demyelination can result from injuries to myelinating cells (oligodendrocytes and Schwann cells). Neurotoxins of this type include lead, which affects Schwann cells possibly by interfering with their Ca^{++} transport, and Cuprizone (biscyclohexanone oxalylhydrazone), which affects oligodendrocytes by its copper chelation, which interfers with adenosine triphosphate formation. Hypocholesterolemic agents such as triparanol, as expected, disrupt myelin sheath because of the high (70%) lipid content of myeline. However, they produce ultrastructural changes in oligodendrocytes before demyelination occurs. Diphtheria toxin demyelinates possibly by affecting both the myelin and the myelinating cells. Ethidium bromide and actinomycin are other examples of demyelinating toxins that act on the myelinating cells.

Myelin Sheath Demyelination can also result from effects on the myelin sheath. This type of effect generally involves a disruption of the membrane structure. Other modes of action include (1) inhibition of carbonic anhydrase or other enzymes involved in ion and water transport, (2) inhibition of enzymes involved in oxidative phosphorylation, and (3) chelation of metals (Cammer, 1980).

Neurotoxins that act directly on the myelin sheath include triethyltin, lysolecithin, isoniazid, cyanate, hexachlorophene, and lead. Most of these toxicants act mainly on the CNS, but lead affects the PNS first. Isoniazid affects the PNS in humans, but in experimental animals its target is the CNS. Acetyl ethyl tetramethyl tetralin (AETT) also causes myelinopathy through a complex mechanism.

The Blood Vessels and Edema

The permeability of the vascular system in the CNS and PNS may be increased by higher blood pressure or lower plasma osmolarity. It may also result from exposure to certain toxins. The greater permeability generally leads to an accumulation of fluids in the extracellular space. Extracellular edema may occur in the CNS or PNS. In addition, a number of neurotoxins are known to induce cellular edema.

Extracellular Edema Lead can damage the endothelial cells and cause extravasation of plasma in the brain, especially in the white matter, which has a greater compliance than the gray matter. That suckling rats are more susceptible to lead has been attributed to the immaturity of the vascular system (Press, 1977). Lead has similar effects in the endoneurium, leading to increased endoneural fluid pressure and demyelination. Organic lead, such as tetraethyl lead, more readily penetrates the barriers and is therefore more toxic in this respect.

Mercury compounds can damage the endothial cells and increase their permeability. Organic arsenicals cause edema and focal hemorrhages in the brain. Tellurium causes edema in the endoneurium. Chronic alcoholism is associated with endoneural edema; the role of the concurrent thiamine deficiency is not known.

Apart from increased vascular permeability, endoneural edema may follow other biologic effects. For example, in experimental animals, a major sign in galactose intoxication is severe endoneural edema in peripheral nerves. Since the edema does not affect dorsal root ganglia, it has been suggested that the polyhydric substance galactitol is synthesized from galactose in the nerves and retained there by the effective PNB (Powell et al., 1979).

Endoneural edema can also result from intramyelinic edema in hexachlorophene intoxication. It may also be associated with wallerian degeneration due to mechanical injury. Mast cells, which accumulate in the distal segment, seem to play an important role (Powell et al., 1980).

Cellular Edema   Various parts of neurons may become edematous following exposure to toxicants. For example, 6-aminonicotinamide affects the perikaryon, cyanide and carbon monoxide affect the axon, and ouabain and methylsulfoxime affect the presynaptic nerve endings.

Edema of astrocytes and oligodendrocytes may be caused by 6-aminonicotinamide. Ouabain can also affect astrocytes. Edema of Schwann cells may be induced by lead, which, as noted above, also may cause extracellular edema.

Triethyltin and isoniazid also cause edema of the myelin sheaths in the CNS. Hexachlorophene induces edema of the myelin sheaths both in the white matter of the brain and in the peripheral nerves.

TESTING PROCEDURES

Neurologic Examinations

These examinations often provide an indication of the site of neurotoxicity; therefore they play a preliminary but important part. Most of these examinations can be performed in humans as well as in animals. The exceptions relate to the determination of *mental state* and many *sensory functions*, which can be more readily assessed in humans. However, appropriate behavioral tests are available for examining animals.

Cranial nerves I through XII have different functions, and their tests therefore vary. For example, tests of the acoustic and optic nerves involve the evaluation of responses to sound and light stimuli.

Motor examination includes inspection of muscles for atrophy, weakness, and fasciculation, which indicate dysfunction of the lower motor neuron, i.e., the anterior horn cells, motor roots, and peripheral nerves. Spasticity is a sign of dysfunction of the upper motor neurons in the brain and their axons down to the spinal cord. Resting tremor is often associated with lesions in the basal ganglia or cerebellum. Intention tremor occurs during voluntary movement and is a manifestation of cerebellar disease.

Reflex examination includes deep tendon reflexes, the functioning of which involves the intrafusal receptors, dorsal root ganglia, anterior horn cells and their axons, neuromuscular junction, and muscle. Damages to any of these structures will cause these reflexes to be absent or hypoactive. On the other hand, when there is upper motor neuron dysfunction, these reflexes will be exaggerated. The Babinski reflex is the most important superficial cutaneous reflex. Abnormal response is an indication of corticospinal dysfunction.

Gait abnormalities may also aid in locating the site of toxicity. For example, lower motor neuron disease causes high-stepping gait. A scissoring, or stiff gait, indicates upper motor neuron lesion. Cerebellar dysfunction results in an ataxic, or reeling gait.

Neurologic signs usually develop rapidly with neuronopathy and myelinopathy but slowly with axonopathy. Axonopathy generally affects both the sensory and motor fibers. On the other hand, neuronopathy affects predominantly the sensory fibers and myelinopathy the motor fibers (Dewar, 1981).

Morphologic Examinations

As described in the section Categories of Neurotoxic Effects, neurotoxins may act on the CNS, the PNS, or both. They may induce lesions in the neuronal perikaryon or its axon, either proximally or distally, the myelinating cells or the myelin sheath itself, the astrocytes, or the endothelial cells. Morphologic examinations are therefore important in establishing the precise site of toxic lesions on an anatomic level. Examinations on cellular and ultrastructural levels often facilitate the diagnosis of the neuropathy and the determination of the mode of action.

Some of the commonly used techniques, along with a list of references, have been provided by Spencer et al. (1980). It is worth noting, however, that damages to endothelial cells can be demonstrated not only by signs of edema (fewer cells and nerve fiber per unit area) but also by increases of the pressure of the intracranial and endoneural fluids as well as by the penetration of tracer substances, such as horseradish peroxidase, through the endothelium.

Electrophysiologic Examinations

Peripheral Nerves A frequently used examination involves the measurement of *motor nerve* conduction velocity (Fullerton, 1966). This can be done on intact animals subjected to chronic or short-term exposure to neurotoxins or on exposed nerves after local application of the toxins. *Sensory nerve* conduction velocity and action potentials have also been measured in the study of neurotoxicity. deJesus et al. (1978) described a procedure using the sural nerve in rats and observed that hexachlorophene decreased the sensory nerve conduction velocity but had no effect on the amplitude of the action potential. On the other hand, zinc pyridinethione reduced the amplitude of the action potential but had no effect on the conduction velocity. Another useful procedure is the measurement of conduction velocity of *slow fibers* (Seppalainen and Hernberg, 1972).

Electromyography This procedure calls for the examination of the electrical activities of a muscle, at rest and when contracted, recorded with the aid of a needle electrode inserted into the muscle. Neurotoxicities may manifest as

(1) abnormal insertional activity, (2) occurrence of spontaneous electrical activity of a resting muscle, and (3) interference pattern of electrical activity of motor units during voluntary muscle contraction. Details of the procedure and interpretation have been described by Goodgold and Eberstein (1977).

Electroencephalography The EEG may be recorded with electrodes placed on the scalp or with electrodes implanted in specific regions in the brain. Johnson (1980) outlined the usefulness of this procedure as well as several others such as sensory evoked potentials, direct electrical stimulation of brain cortex, the absolute refractory period, and the stimulus strength-duration testing.

Biochemical Examinations

As noted above, the nervous system depends almost entirely on glucose metabolism for its energy. Since the enzyme systems involved in glucose metabolism are often the target of toxicants, their activities merit investigation, as do the systems involved in ion transport, which is vital to nerve impluse conduction. Protein synthesis is impaired by a number of neurotoxicants. The compositions of various subcellular structures and myelin sheath are also fruitful subjects of biochemical examination. The migration of radiolabeled materials along axons and transneurally is another useful procedure. Other biochemical parameters include the levels of neurotransmitters at specific sites in the nervous system and the binding of neurotransmitter receptors by the use of agonists and antagonists (Damstra and Bondy, 1980; Dewar, 1981).

NERVE CELL CULTURES

Apart from the various testing procedures described above, cells from fetal brain, the spinal cord, and dorsal root ganglia can be mechanically or enzymatically segregated and grown in suitable culture media. The cells grow and differentiate in the media. They can be subjected to electrophysiologic, morphologic, and biochemical examinations to assess the effects of neurotoxicants (Nelson, 1978; Trapp and Richelson, 1980).

BEHAVIORAL STUDIES

There is a large body of information on behavioral toxicology, resulting from a widespread feeling that behavior is a subtle and sensitive indicator of toxicity. However, this view has been questioned, for example, by Norton (1980b), who stated: "Scientific data supporting this view are not only scanty but the available evidence often flatly contradicts this assumption." In the hope that improved testing procedures would increase the sensitivity and utility of this approach in neurotoxicology, this branch of neurotoxicology will undoubtedly grow. A few highlights of this subject are presented below.

Testing Procedures

The tests involve two types of responses: (1) unconditioned responses, which are either emitted (spontaneous) or elicited (reflex), and (2) conditioned responses, which may be considered as either "classic conditioning" (Pavlov) or operant conditioning (Skinner). The extent of training of the experimental animals required and the neurobehavioral function to be assessed are also useful criteria for classification of the tests.

Simple Tests Tilson et al. (1980) listed tests that require little or no prior training of the experimental animals (rats and mice) (see Table 17-1).

More Involved Tests The tests listed in Table 17-2 require extended or special training, frequent evaluation, and/or manipulation of motivational factors.

Table 17-1 Examples of Primary Level Neurobehavioral Tests for Rats or Mice

Neurobehavioral function	Behavioral test
Sensory	
Visual, olfactory, somatosensory, auditory	Localization
Pain	Tail flick
Orientation in space	Negative geotaxis
Motor	
Spontaneous activity	Activity in Automex
Muscular weakness	Forelimb grip; hindlimb extensor
Fatiguability	Swim endurance
Tremor	Frequency of occurrence
Cognitive-associative	
Learning and retention	One-way avoidance; step-through passive avoidance
Affective-emotional	
Responsiveness	Startle to air puff; emergence in a novel environment
Physiologic-consummatory	
Thermoregulation	Body weight; food and water ingestion; core temperature

From Tilson et al., 1980. (Reproduced with permission of Peter S. Spencer, Editor.)

Table 17-2 Examples of Secondary Level Neurobehavioral Tests for Rats or Mice

Neurobehavioral function	Behavioral test
Sensory	
Visual, auditory, olfactory	Operant psychophysics
Gustatory	Taste discrimination
Somatosensory	T-maze discrimination
Orientation in space	T-maze discrimination
Pain	Operant titration
Motor	
Spontaneous activity	Diurnal cyclicity; patterning
Muscular strength	Operant response force
Tremor	Spectral analysis
Cognitive-associative	
Learning and retention	Autoshaping; temporal discriminating; repeated acquisition
Affective-emotional	
CNS excitability	Brain self-stimulation; aversion thresholds
Physiologic-consummatory	
Thermoregulation	Diurnal patterning; cyclicity; preference

From Tilson et al., 1980. (Reproduced with permission of Peter S. Spencer, Editor.)

Procedures to Enhance Sensitivity Because of the large functional reserve of the brain, focal damages may not result in any overt brain dysfunction. Such damages, however, may be demonstrated clinically with the use of *provocative* tests. These involve administering sodium amobarbital, raising body temperature, or lowering blood pH with the intravenous infusion of ammonium chloride (Lehrer, 1974).

Animals Apart from rats and mice, other animals such as pigeons, cats, dogs, and monkeys are also commonly used, with testing procedures similar to those listed above.

Results

Behavioral tests have been extensively used in assessing the neurotoxicity of solvents, heavy metals (especially lead and mercury), pesticides, and certain CNS drugs (alcohol, amphetamines). The results have been reviewed and summarized in the proceedings of a NIOSH workshop (1974). Reviews of behavioral studies on certain food additives in humans and animals have been prepared, respectively, by Weiss et al. (1979) and Butcher (1979).

EVALUATION

In view of the wide range of toxic effects on the nervous system, as outlined above, there is clearly need for a battery of tests for the evaluation of neurotoxins. It is also worth noting that the choice of animal species is critical in eliciting certain types of toxicity, such as delayed neurotoxicity. Furthermore, the nature of the toxicity on the nervous system, as on other organs, can vary according to the duration of exposure. For example, n-hexane and TOCP produce, after acute exposure, narcosis, a CNS effect, but they induce axonopathy after repeated exposures.

The significance of a neurotoxic effect depends on its reversibility. In general, irreversible effects are more serious than reversible ones. The site of the effect also plays an important role. There are areas in the nervous system more critical to physiologic function than others. In addition, focal damages in areas with abundant functional reserve are likely to be less serious.

In evaluating toxicologic results, it is essential to ensure their validity. In other words, efforts must be made to rule out chance observations, artifacts stemming from improper testing procedures, and others. These precautions are also applicable to neurotoxicology, perhaps behavioral toxicology in particular.

The behavioral effects are especially susceptible to endogenous and environmental variations. For example, Norton (1980b) reported data to indicate a large variability of results both between animals of the same species and within variations of the same animal at different times. It is therefore important to adhere to proper experimental procedures, e.g., sufficiently large number of animals, rigorously controlled experimental environment, statistical analysis of results.

To facilitate proper interpretation of behavioral effects of neurotoxic agents, Tilson et al. (1979) recommended validation with agents that are known to produce specific effects. For example, they recommended the use of triethyltin in studies involving demyelination and methyl mercury and inorganic lead in studies involving mixed central and peripheral neuropathies.

REFERENCES

Asbury, A. K., and Brown, M. J. (1980) The evolution of structural changes in distal axonopathies. In: *Experimental and Clinical Neurotoxicology*, pp. 179–192. Eds. P. S. Spencer and H. H. Schaumberg, Baltimore: William & Wilkins.

Blatteis, C. M. (1981) The newer putative central neurotransmitters: Roles in thermoregulation. *Fed. Proc.* 40:2735–2700.

Butcher, R. (1979) A survey of early tests for the developmental psychotoxicity of food additives and related compounds. Proceedings of the Fifth FDA Science Symposium. Rockville, Maryland: U.S. Food and Drug Administration.

Cammer, W. (1980) Toxic demyelination: Biochemical studies and hypothetical mechanisms. In: *Experimental and Clinical Neurotoxicology*, pp. 239–256. Eds. P. S. Spencer and H. H. Schaumberg. Baltimore: Williams & Wilkins.

Cavanagh, J. B. (1977) Metabolic mechanisms of neurotoxicity caused by mercury. In: *Neurotoxicology*. Eds. L. Roizin, H. Shiraki, and N. Grcevic. New York: Raven Press.

Cho, E. S., Spencer, P. S., and Jortner, B. S. (1980). Doxorubicin. In: *Experimental and Clinical Neurotoxicology*, pp. 440–455. Eds. P. S. Spencer and H. H. Schaumberg. Baltimore: Williams & Wilkins.

Crapper, D. R., and DeBoni, U. (1980) Aluminum. In: *Experimental and Clinical Neurotoxicology*, pp. 326–335. Eds. P. S. Spencer and H. H. Schaumberg. Baltimore: Williams & Wilkins.

Damstra, T., and Bondy, S. C. (1980) The current status and future of biochemical assays for neurotoxicity. In *Experimental and Clinical Neurotoxicology*, pp. 820–833. Eds. P. S. Spencer and H. H. Schaumberg. Baltimore: Williams & Wilkins.

Davis, C. S., and Richardson, R. J. (1980) Organophosphorus compounds. In: *Experimental and Clinical Neurotoxicology*, pp. 527–544. Eds. P. S. Spencer and H. H. Schaumberg. Baltimore: Williams & Wilkins.

deJesus, C. P. V., Towfighi, J., and Snyder, J. R. (1978) Sural nerve conduction study in the rat: A new technique for studying experimental neuropathies. *Muscle Nerve* 1:162–167.

Dewar, A. J. (1981) Neurotoxicity testing—with particular reference to biochemical methods. In: *Testing for Toxicity*. Ed. J. W. Gorrod. London: Taylor & Francis.

Fullerton, P. M., and Barnes, J. M. (1966) Peripheral neuropathy in rats produced by acrylamide. *Brit. J. Ind. Med.* 23:210–221.

Goodgold, J., and Eberstein, A. (1977) *Electrodiagnosis of Neuromuscular Diseases*. Baltimore: Williams & Wilkins.

Griffin, J. W., and Price, D. L. (1980) Proximal axonopathies induced by toxic chemicals. In: *Experimental and Clinical Neurotoxicology*, pp. 161–178. Eds. P. S. Spencer and H. H. Schaumberg. Baltimore: Williams & Wilkins.

Jacobs, J. M. (1980) Vascular permeability and neural injury. In: *Experimental and Clinical Neurotoxicology*, pp. 102–117. Eds. P. S. Spencer and H. H. Schaumberg. Baltimore: Williams & Wilkins.

Jacobs, J. M., Carmichael, N., and Cavanagh, J. B. (1975) Ultrastructural changes in the dorsal root and trigeminal ganglia of rats poisoned with methyl mercury. *Neuropathol. Appl. Neurobiol.* 1:1–19.

Jacobs, J. M., Carmichael, N., and Cavanagh, J. B. (1977) Ultrastructural studies in the nervous system of rabbits poisoned with methyl mercury. *Toxicol. Appl. Pharmacol.* 39:249–261.

Johnson, B. L. (1980) Electrophysiological methods in neurotoxicity testing. In: *Experimental and Clinical Neurotoxicology*, pp. 726–742. Eds. P. S. Spencer and H. H. Schaumberg. Baltimore: Williams & Wilkins.

Lehrer, G. M. (1974) Measurement of minimal brain dysfunction. In: *Behavior Toxicology*. Eds. C. Xintaras, B. L. Johnson and I. de Groot. Washington, D.C.: National Institute for Occupational Safety and Health.

Narahashi, T. (1980) Nerve membrane as a target of environmental toxicants. In: *Experimental and Clinical Neurotoxicology*, pp. 225–238. Eds. P. S. Spencer and H. H. Schaumberg. Baltimore: Williams & Wilkins.

Nelson, P. G. (1978) Neuronal cell cultures as toxicologic test systems. *Environ. Health Perspect.* 26:125–133.

NIOSH (1974) *Behavioral Toxicology*. Eds. C. Xintaras, B. L. Johnson, and I. de Groot. Washington, D.C.: National Institute for Occupational Safety and Health.

Norton, S. (1980a) Toxic responses of the central nervous system. In: *Casarett and Doull's Toxicology*. Eds. J. Doull, C. D. Klaassen, and M. O. Amdur. New York: Macmillan.

Norton, S. (1980b) Behavioral toxicology: A critical appraisal. In: *The Scientific Basis of Toxicity Assessment*. Ed. H. R. Witschi. Amsterdam: Elsevier/North Holland.

OECD (1984) Delayed neurotoxicity of organophosphorus substances. In: *Guidelines for Testing Chemicals*. Paris: Organization for Economic Co-operation and Development.

Olney, J. W. (1980) Excitotoxic mechanisms of neurotoxicity. In: *Experimental and Clinical Neurotoxicology*, pp. 272–294. Eds. P. S. Spencer and H. H. Schaumberg. Baltimore: Williams & Wilkins.

Politis, M. J., Pellegrino, R. G., and Spencer, P. S. (1980) Ultrastructural studies of the dying back process. V. Axonal neurofilaments accumulate at sites of 2,5-hexadione application: Evidence for nerve fiber dysfunction in experimental neuropathy. *J. Neurocytol.* 9:505–516.

Powell, H. C., Myers, R. R., and Costello, M. L. (1979) Endoneurial fluid pressure and pathologic findings in galactose neuropathy. *J. Neuropathol. Exp. Neurol.* 38:335.

Powell, H. C., Myers, R. R., and Lampert, P. W. (1980) Edema in neurotoxic injury. In: *Experimental and Clinical Neurotoxicology*, pp. 118–138. Eds. P. S. Spencer and H. H. Schaumberg. Baltimore: Williams & Wilkins.

Press, M. F. (1977) Lead encephalopathy in neonatal Long-Evans rats: Morphologic studies. *J. Neuropathol. Exp. Neurol.* 36:169–193.

Savolainen, H. (1977) Some aspects of the mechanism by which industrial solvents produce neurotoxic effects. *Chem. Biol. Interact.* 18:1–10.

Schield, L. K., Griffin, J. W., Drachman, D. B., and Price, D. L. (1977) Retrograde axonal transport: A direct method for measurement of rate. *Neurology* 27:393.

Schoental, R., and Cavanagh, J. B. (1977) Mechanisms involved in the "dying-back" process—an hypothesis implicating coenzymes. *Neuropathol. Appl. Neurobiol.* 3:145.

Seppalainen, A. M., and Hernberg, S. (1972) Sensitive technique for detecting subclinical lead neuropathy. *Br. J. Ind. Med.* 29:443–449.

Spencer, P. S., Bischoff, M. C., and Schaumberg, H. H. (1980) Neuropathological methods for the detection of neurotoxic disease. In: *Experimental and Clinical Neurotoxicology*, pp. 743–757. Eds. P. S. Spencer and H. H. Schaumberg. Baltimore: Williams & Wilkins.

Spencer, P. S., Sabri, M. I., Schaumberg, H. H., and Moore, C. (1979) Does a defect in energy metabolism in the nerve fiber cause axonal degeneration in polyneuropathies? *Ann. Neurol.* 5:501–507.

Tilson, H. A., Cabe, P. A., and Burne, T. A. (1980) Behavioral procedures for the assessment of neurotoxicity. In: *Experimental and Clinical Neurotoxicology*, pp. 758–766. Eds. P. C. Spencer and H. H. Schaumberg. Baltimore: Williams & Wilkins.

Tilson, H. A., Mitchell, C. L., and Cabe, P. A. (1979) Screening for neurobehavioral toxicity: The need for and examples of validation of testing procedures. *Neurobehav. Toxicol.* 1(Suppl. 1):137–148.

Trapp, B. D., and Richelson, E. (1980) Usefulness for neurotoxicology of rotation-mediated aggregating cell cultures. In: *Experimental and Clinical Toxicology*, pp. 803–819. Eds. P. S. Spencer and H. H. Schaumberg. Baltimore: Williams & Wilkins.

Weiss, B., Cox, C., Young, M., Margen, S., and Williams, J. H. (1979) *Neurobehav. Toxicol.* 1(Suppl. 1):149–156.

Chapter 18

Reproductive, Cardiac, and Immune Systems

Reproductive System

INTRODUCTION

Reproductive Process

The process starts with gametogenesis. In the female animal, oogenesis involves the formation of primary oocytes from the primordial germ cells (oogonia) through mitosis. This development takes place during the fetal period and ceases at birth. Primary oocytes divide by meiosis to form secondary oocytes just before they are ovulated.

On the other hand, spermatogenesis starts with gonocytes during the fetal period, and these cells are transformed to spermatogonia after birth. Spermatogonia remain dormant until puberty, when proliferative activity begins again. Some of the spermatogonia multiply to form additional spermatogonia while others mature to spermatozoa. There are three intermediate stages. Spermatogonia divide by mitosis to form primary spermatocytes, which divide by meiosis to form secondary spermatocytes. These in turn divide by meiosis to form spermatids. Finally spermatids become spermatozoa by metamorphosis. The entire process is continuous, and the time required for spermatogonia to become spermatozoa is about 60 days (Fig. 18-1).

Fertilization requires not only functional ovum and spermatozoa but also effective delivery of the sperm and proper milieu. The conceptus, the fertilized ovum, is then implanted in uterus and develops through embryonic and fetal stages. At the end of the gestational period, parturition takes place. The pups are suckled until weaning. They then grow and mature to start the reproductive process again, thus completing a reproductive cycle.

Pharmacokinetics

Throughout the reproductive cycle, toxicants can interfere with the various events and processes enumerated above. They may act directly on the reproductive system or the conceptus or indirectly via certain endocrine organs. Before chemicals act directly, they must reach the target organs in sufficiently high concentration. This concentration may be higher or lower than that in the blood.

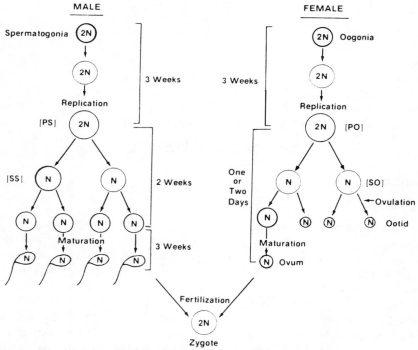

Figure 18-1 Gametogenesis and fertilization. 2N, diploid; N, haploid; PS, primary spermatocyte; SS, secondary spermatocyte; PO, primary oocyte; SO, secondary oocyte. (From Brusick, 1980, by permission.)

For example, with DDT, the concentration is almost 80 times higher in the ovary than in the plasma. A number of other substances have also been shown to penetrate the oocyte, oviduct, uterine fluid, and blastocyst (Fabro, 1978).

Toxicity of chemicals on the testis is influenced by the blood-testis barrier (BTB) and by activities of certain enzymes (Lee and Dixon, 1978). The BTB is a complex multicellular system composed of both myoid cells surrounding the seminiferous tubules and several layers of spermatogenic cells in the tubules. Thus they form a barrier, although much less effective than the blood-brain barrier. The penetration rate of chemicals into the testis is proportional to their molecular weights and their partition coefficients.

Testis contains both activating and detoxicating enzyme systems. These two enzyme systems, as noted in Chapter 3, are capable of, respectively, increasing and decreasing the toxicities of chemicals. Furthermore, there is an efficient DNA repair system in the premeiotic spermatogenic cells, but there is none in spermatids nor in spermatozoa. Mutations can therefore be induced by electrophilic substances.

TOXIC EFFECTS

Many chemicals adversely affect spermatogenesis and cause testicular atrophy. These include food colors (e.g., Oil Yellow AB and Oil Yellow OB) (Allmark et al., 1955), pesticides (e.g., DBCP), metals (e.g., lead and cadmium), and organic solvents. A variety of other chemicals affect the testis, such as steroid hormones, alkylating agents, cyclohexylamine, and hexachlorophene (Dixon, 1980). Hypotensive drugs such as guanethidine (like thalidomide), can induce nonpregnancy by interfering with seminal emission rather than by any direct effect on the fetus (Palmer, 1976).

A variety of chemicals may be toxic to female reproductive functions (Dixon, 1980). Certain chemicals affect the oocyte, others (e.g., haloperidol) prevent implantation or affect the development and growth of the conceptus. For example, nicotine and DDT lower fetal weight in rabbits (Fabro, 1978). Some chemicals (e.g., spironolactone) have various effects on reproductive functions, such as interference with ovulation and implantation and retardation of development of the sex organs of the offspring (Nagi and Virgo, 1982).

The toxic effects that are specifically related to the production of congenital anomalies are dealt with in Chapter 11, Teratogenesis.

ROUTINE TESTING

Multigeneration Reproduction Studies

Procedure In general, rats are the animal of choice. A minimum of 20 females and 10 males are placed in each of three dose groups and a control group. The doses are so selected that the high dose will produce some minimal toxic signs but will not result in a mortality greater than 10%. The low dose will not induce any observable effect.

Prior to breeding, the males are dosed throughout the period of spermatogenesis (60–80 days) and the females are dosed throughout the development of the ova (16 days). Dosing of the females is continued through the gestation and lactation periods. The test chemical should be administered by a route that most closely resembles the human exposure condition.

To determine the potential effect of the chemical on the reproductive function of the offspring (F_1), a second generation offspring (F_2) is bred and reared to reproductive maturity.

Observations and Examinations The adult animals are observed for the body weight, food consumption, general appearance, estrus cycle, and mating behavior. In addition, the fertility and nesting and nursing behaviors are also noted. Half of the maternal rats are killed on day 13 of gestation for examination of corpora lutea, implantations, and resorptions (Jones, 1981; Morton, 1981).

The other half of the maternal rats are allowed to deliver their pups. The pups are examined for litter size, number of stillborn, sex distribution, and congenital anomalies. In addition, the viability and pup weight are recorded at birth, on day 4, and at weaning, and preferably also on day 12 or 14. Auditory and visual functions and behavior are also examined for subtle congenital defects.

An appropriate number of males and females are randomly selected from all generations and examined by gross necropsy and histopathology, especially with respect to the reproductive organs.

Additional details and references to the multigeneration reproduction studies are provided by Dixon (1980) and in the EPA test guidelines (EPA, 1982).

Evaluation From the data described, the following reproductive indices can be derived (EPA, 1978):

1   Fertility index: the percentage of matings resulting in pregnancy
2   Gestation index: the percentage of pregnancies resulting in the birth of live litters
3   Viability index: the percentage of live pups that survive 4 days or longer
4   Lactation index: the percentage of pups alive on day 4 that survive 21 days or longer

Other indicators include (1) mating index (the percentage of estrus cycles that had matings), (2) male fertility index (the percentage of males exposed to fertile nonpregnant females that resulted in pregnancies), (3) female fertility index (the percentage of females exposed to fertile males that resulted in pregnancies), and (4) 12- or 14-day survival indices.

Multigeneration reproductive study can reveal a variety of toxic effects on the reproductive function as well as on the conceptus. However, nonspecific response (e.g., nonpregnancy) is common. It may follow unusual routes of administering the chemical, such as inhalation, topical application to the eye or nose, and parenteral administration. Excessive handling may also disturb the normal reproductive function. A number of other interfering factors are discussed by Palmer (1976).

The pathologic examination may reveal suppression of spermatogenesis, advanced rates of follicle atresia, and ovulatory or meiotic failure.

Adjunct Tests To save time and expenses, the males of the parent generation (F_0) used in the multigeneration study may be used in a dominant lethal test, and a second litter of the first generation offspring (F_{1b}) may be bred for a teratogenicity study.

OTHER TESTS

The effects revealed in multigeneration reproduction studies outlined above may result from paternal, maternal, or fetal exposure. Thus, additional tests are often conducted to establish the cause of the effect. A few such tests are outlined below.

Perinatal and *postnatal* studies are often conducted to determine effects on late development of the offspring. The procedure is essentially the same as that of the multigeneration study, except that only the females are treated and their treatment covers only the last third of gestation and throughout lactation. The litter data, as described above, are recorded and evaluated (Palmer, 1976).

Analysis of *semen* is useful in epidemiologic and animal studies. The sperm count and their motility, survival, and morphology often provide information on toxic effects on testis (Eliasson, 1978).

The *perfused male reproductive tracts* have been shown to be useful models in studying the effects of chemicals on the secretion and accumulation of androgens (Bardin et al., 1978).

Brackett (1978) described a procedure using *in vitro fertilized ova* in the study of toxic effects by observing development of the ova.

Heart

GENERAL CONSIDERATIONS

The heart is a vital organ in the body. Although it is not a common target organ, it can be damaged by a variety of chemicals. They act either directly on the myocardium or indirectly through the nervous system or blood vessels. A list of such chemicals, as compiled by Van Stee (1980), is reproduced in Table 18-1.

Table 18-1 Cardiotoxic Drugs and Chemicals

Electrophysiologic mechanisms:
Cardiotonic drugs	Local anesthetics
Phenytoin (diphenylhydantoin)	Emetine
Tricyclic antidepressants	Chlordimeform
Clofibrate	Contrast media
Lithium	Antimalarial drugs
Propylene glycol	Calcium antagonists

Nonspecific myocardial depression:
Lipid-soluble, organic compounds	Antimicrobial antibiotics
Myocardial depressant factor	Carbromide, carbromal

Interference with nucleic acid metabolism and protein synthesis:
Antineoplastic drugs

Cardiomyopathy:
Allylamine	Adrenergic agonists
Furazolidone	Methysergide
Ethanol	Vasodilators
Cobalt	

Involvement with lipid metabolism:
High cholesterol diet	Brominated vegetable oils
Rapeseed oil	

Miscellaneous:
Phenothiazines

Source: Van Stee, 1980.

The heart is mainly composed of myocardial cells, each measuring about 15 × 80 μm. Unlike skeletal muscle cells, each of which is innervated, only a portion of the heart muscle cells are innervated. However, these cells are joined, at their ends, to each other by the nexus. It has low resistance and thus allows rapid transmission of electrical stimulus from one cell to the next. These characteristics are essential to the programmed sequence of contraction of different parts of the heart.

The myocardium is different from skeletal muscles also in that there is less contractile material (50% vs. 80%) but much more mitochondrial material (35% vs. 2%). Mitochondria evidently play an important role in the cardiac contractility and are a common subcellular target of cardiotoxicity.

Myocardial contraction involves the liberation of energy from oxidative metabolism, conservation of the energy by adenosine triphosphate and creatine phosphate and utilization of the energy by contractile proteins. The most vulnerable mechanisms probably include the utilization of energy and intracellular movement of calcium ion (Merin, 1978).

TOXIC EFFECTS

Cardiomyopathy

The usual toxic effects of cobalt are polycythemia, goiter, and signs of gastrointestinal irritation such as vomiting and diarrhea. However, its inclusion in beer as a foam stabilizer caused a number of serious and fatal cases of cardio-myopathy (Morin and Daniel, 1967). Subsequent studies showed that there is also intramitochondrial accumulation of calcium. The toxicity of cobalt on the heart was greatly enhanced by malnutrition, especially the deficiency of certain amino acids. Among the beer drinkers, this condition existed because of the large caloric intake of beer. It was also noted that cobalt ions depressed oxygen uptake and interfered with cardiac energy metabolism in the tricarboxylic acid cycle, as thiamine deficiency does (Grice, 1972).

A number of adrenergic β-receptor agonists, notably isoproterenol, and vasodilating antihypertensive drugs, e.g., hydralazine and diazoxide, are capable of inducing myocardial necrosis. The former chemicals have direct adrenergic effects, whereas the antihypertensive drugs exert adrenergic effects via the in-duced hypotension. These effects produced an augmented transmembrane cal-cium influx, which in turn causes an increase in the rate and force of contrac-tion. This, along with the concomitant hypotension, results in hypoxia. The hypoxia and the calcium deposits in the mitochondria cause disintegration of organelles and sarcolemma (Balazs and Ferrans, 1978; Balazs et al., 1981).

Interference with Nucleic Acid Synthesis

The anthracycline antibiotics doxorubicin and daunorubicin are effective anti-neoplastic drugs. However, they produce hypotension, tachycardia and arrhyth-mias acutely. More prolonged administration causes degeneration and atrophy of cardiac muscle cells and interstitial edema and fibrosis. The likely mode of action is the binding of these antibiotics to mitochondrial and nuclear DNA, which in turn interfers with synthesis of RNA and protein. This effect on the heart is important because the half-life of the contractile proteins is short (1-2 weeks). Other possible mechanisms of action include (1) inhibition of Q en-zymes, (2) peroxidation of membrane lipids, and (3) hypotension resulting from release of histamine (Van Stee, 1980).

Arrhythmias

A number of fluorocarbons are capable of producing cardiac arrhythmias. This effect is mediated by a sensitization of the heart to epinephrine, depression of contractility, reduction of coronary blood flow, and reflex increase in sympa-thetic and vagal impulses to the heart following irritation of mucosa in the respiratory tract (Aviado, 1978).

Tricyclic antidepressants also can cause cardiac arrhythmias. These effects are likely the result of imbalances within the autonomic regulatory system of the heart. Propylene glycol, a common solvent, can convert ventricular tachy-cardia induced by deslanoside into ventricular fibrillation (Van Stee, 1980).

Myocardial Depression

A number of lipid-soluble organic compounds, such as general anesthetics, depress cardiac contractility. The probable mechanism of action is a nonspecific expansion of various cellular membranes by the insertion of chemically indifferent molecules in the hydrophobic regions of integral proteins and membrane phospholipids.

The aminoglycoside antibiotics, such as neomycin and streptomycin, cause hypotension through depression of cardiac contractility. However, the mechanism of action appears to be related to an inhibition of a portion of Ca^{2+} bound to superficial membrane sites (Adams et al., 1978).

Miscellaneous

Rapeseed oil, a common cooking oil in many parts of the world, causes accumulation of lipid globules in heart muscles in rats. This effect was attributed to the high content of erucic acid in rapeseed oil. Brominated vegetable oils, used in adjusting the density of flavoring oils and in enhancing cloudy stability in beverages, induce biochemical and morphologic changes in cardiac myofibrils. The coloring Brown F.K. also produces severe morphologic changes in the heart muscles (Grice, 1972).

TESTING PROCEDURES

Cardiotoxicity can be studied in intact normal animals, in animals with specific pathologic conditions, or in isolated hearts.

Normal Animals

A variety of examinations for cardiotoxicity can be performed on animals in conventional toxicity studies. These include blood pressure, heart rate, and electrocardiography. Functional tests, such as swimming till exhaustion, have been suggested. After necropsy, the organ weight is often determined. Gross, light, and, in particular, electron microscopic examinations are valuable. Biochemical studies of the myocardium and of the blood are also useful. Additional details and references to these tests are provided by Van Stee (1980).

Animals with Pathologic Conditions

The hearts of rabbits fed a diet containing 2% cholesterol become atherosclerotic. These hearts are more susceptible to myocardial ischemia (Lee et al., 1978). Other models, such as infarcted myocardium, cardiomyopathic hamster, obesity, and drug interaction models have been briefly described and referenced by Van Stee (1980).

Isolated Heart

The isolated, perfused heart is a common model for studying the effects of drugs on the strength and rate of heart contractions and the rate of coronary flow. It has also been used to detect the cardiac effects of toxicants. For example, Toy et al. (1976) have shown that certain halogenated alkanes depressed the peak left ventricular pressure as well as the rate of increase of that pressure. The isolated atrium and cultured heart cells have also been used in the study of cardiotoxicity (Adams et al., 1978; Sperelakis, 1978).

Evaluation

The cardiotoxicity of chemicals is not readily detected in conventional toxicity studies. For example, the toxic effects of cobalt and the anthracycline antibiotics on the heart were reproduced in animal experiments only after they were detected in humans first. Negative results therefore do not necessarily exclude potential cardiotoxicity.

To demonstrate such toxicity, specific testing procedures may be required. These procedures usually mimic the clinical conditions. For example, intermittent administration of the anthracycline antibiotics was necessary to elicit the cardiotoxicity; presumably continuous treatment caused the animals to die from other toxic effects before heart lesions developed. The toxicity of adrenergic β-receptor agonists is best detected in acute studies; the effects of prolonged treatment may be masked by tolerance development. The effect of cobalt on the heart is more readily revealed when the animals are on a protein- and vitamin-deficient diet (Balazs and Ferrans, 1978).

Immune System

GENERAL CONSIDERATIONS

The immune system serves an important role in the body's defense against infections by viruses, bacteria, fungi, and unicellular and multicellular parasites as well as against neoplastic cells.

It is now established that a variety of chemicals can impair the function of the system. A number of chemicals may induce hypersensitivity reactions. The site of such reactions are mainly confined to the respiratory tract and the skin, as described in Chapters 12 and 15.

COMPONENTS OF THE SYSTEM

It consists of a network of organs including the bone marrow, thymus, spleen, and lymph nodes. From these organs, a variety of lymphocytes and other cells with different immune functions are derived.

T Cells

Certain stem cells in the bone marrow pass through the thymus and become T cells (T lymphocytes). These cells enter the blood and constitute 70% of the circulating lymphocytes. Some settle in thymus-dependent areas of the spleen and lymph nodes. These small and medium-sized lymphocytes have a life-span of 15–20 years.

On contact with macrophage-processed antigen, the T cells undergo proliferation and differentiation. Some of these "committed T cells" become *activated* and responsible for mediating cellular immunity. Others become T *memory* cells, which can be activated by combining with antigens; still others by becoming *helper* or *suppressor* cells serve to regulate the production of antibodies by B cells.

The activated T cells react either directly with cell-membrane–associated antigens or by releasing various soluble factors known as lymphokines. There are a large number of lymphokines, the most important of which are (1) mitogenic factor, (2) migration inhibition factor, (3) skin reactive factor, (4) interferon, (5) lymphotoxin, (6) macrophage activation factor, and (7) chemotactins that attract eosinophils, macrophages, neutrophils, and other lymphocytes (Cohen and McCluskey, 1979).

B Cells

Other stem cells undergo changes in tissues having the function of the bursa of Fabricius (i.e., bone marrow; the lymphoid tissues in the gut such as the appendix, cecum, and the Peyer's patches) to become B cells (B lymphocytes). They enter the blood to constitute 30% of the lymphocytes. Their life-span is only 15 days.

The primary immune response is initiated by the contact of antigen with B cells, which then differentiate and proliferate. Some of these become *memory* cells, which retain the surface immunoglobulin receptors, whereas others become *plasma* cells. The latter type of cells are mature and capable of synthesizing small amounts of IgM immunoglobulins. Exposure of the memory cells to the same antigen at a later time results in the secondary immune response. This response differs from the primary type in that not only do all the processes proceed much more rapidly but the immunoglobulins are of the IgG class and in greater quantities. Other B cells remain in the bone marrow and become IgA-producing cells. The differentiation of the B cells to plasma cells is regulated by the helper and suppressor T cells.

Other Components

Other lymphocytic cells lack the characteristic surface markers of the T cells and the B cells, but they participate in the immune system functions. These are the *natural killer* cells (NK) and the null cells. The former are active in immune cytotoxic functions, whereas the latter are active in antibody-dependent cell-mediated cytotoxicity. A comprehensive list of the properties of these two types of cells has been compiled (Stutman et al., 1981).

Macrophages, like lymphocytes, are also derived from the stem cell pool in the bone marrow. After their release, they appear in the bloodstream as monocytes and in the tissues as histiocytes. On contact with a foreign body, they engulf the foreign body and become activated macrophages. These cells are rich in cytoplasmic hydrolytic enzymes. Most bacterial cells are readily digested by these enzymes. Macrophages can also be activated, as noted above, by certain lymphokines produced by T cells. Polymorphonuclear leukocytes, like macrophages, are also active in phagocytosis. Opsonizing antibodies and complement factors enhance this activity.

Complement is a group of circulating plasma proteins that become enzymes after splitting from their natural inhibitors. Such activation of the complement is generally initiated by the antigen-antibody complex. The antigen can be erythrocyte, bacteria, virus, or other cells, and the antibody can be IgG_1, IgG_2, IgG_3, or IgM. The complement serves to amplify and extend immunologic interactions.

TOXIC SUBSTANCES

A variety of substances have been found to affect the immune system (see Dean et al., 1979). They may be placed in the following categories:

1 Antineoplastic drugs: cyclophosphoramide, nitrogen mustards, 6-mercaptopurine, azathioprine, methotrexate, 5-fluorouracil, actinomycin, doxorubicin
2 Heavy metals, organometals, etc.: lead, cadmium, nickel, chromium, methyl mercury, di-*N*-octyltin dichloride, di-*N*-butyltin dichloride, sodium arsenite and arsenate, and arsenic trioxide
3 Pesticides: DDT, dieldrin, carbaryl, carbofuran, methylparathion, maneb, chlordane, hexachlorobenzene (HCB)
4 Halogenated hydrocarbons: PCB, polybrominated biphenyls (PBB), TCDD, trichloroethylene, chloroform, pentachlorophenol
5 Miscellaneous compounds: benzo[a]pyrene, methylcholanthrene, diethylstilbestrol, benzene, glucocorticoids

A number of these substances act by covalent binding with critical macromolecules, thereby inhibiting cell proliferation or otherwise interfering with cellular functions.

The effects of toxicants on the immune system are complex, as shown in Table 18-2, with data from Dean et al. (1982a).

Table 18-2 Effects of In Vivo Exposure to Chemicals on Immune Function and Host Resistance

Parameters	DES	BaP	TPA
Resistance to *Listeria* challenge	D	NE	I
Resistance to tumor challenge	D	NE	D
Trichinella expulsion	D	D	NE
Thymus weight	D	NE	D
Delayed hypersensitivity	D	NE	NE
Lymphocyte responses[*]	D	D[†]	D
T-cell quantification	D	—	D
Spontaneous lymphocyte cytotoxicity	NE	NE	D
Antibody plague response	D	D	D
Immunoglobulins M, G, and A levels	NE	NE	D
Macrophage phagocytosis	I	NE	I
Macrophage cytostasis	I	NE	I
RES clearance time	I	NE	I
Bone marrow cellularity[‡]	D	D	NE

Source: Data from Dean et al., 1982. (© 1982, American Society for Pharmacology and Experimental Therapeutics)

DES, diethylstilbestrol; BaP (benzo[a] pyrene); TPA (12-o-tetradecanoylphorbol-13-o-acetate); D, decreased; I, increased; NE, no effect; —, not tested.

[*]Lymphocyte responses to phytohemagglutinin, concanavalin A, lipopolysaccharide and mixed lymphocyte culture.

[†]Decreased, except the response to mixed lymphocyte culture.

[‡]Colony-forming units—multipotent cells and granulocyte/macrophage progenators.

TESTING PROCEDURES

A large number of tests have been developed to study the immunotoxicologic effect of chemicals. While more investigation is required to define the optimum conditions and procedures and to compare their relative significance in terms of human health, the following tests appear to be in common use (Dean et al., 1982a).

Immunocompetence Tests in Intact Animals

These tests are designed to study the effects of chemicals on host resistance/susceptibility to bacterial, viral, and parasitic diseases as well as to bacterial endotoxins and tumor cells. In general, mice are used because of the large number of animals required.

The test chemical is given to the animals by an appropriate route, preferably mimicking the human exposure. Usually three dose groups plus a control group are included in the test. The duration of the dosing is generally 14 or 90 days. After this pretreatment, the animals are given a suitable quantity of the challenging agent. The quantity of the agent is selected on the basis that 10-20%

of the mortality or morbidity is induced in the control animals. Increased mortality or morbidity indicates decreased host resistance.

Tumor cells used in such tests include those induced by chemicals (e.g., methylcholanthrene) or by virus (e.g., Moloney sarcoma virus).

Various infectious agents are used: (1) *viruses*, including encephalomyocarditis virus and *Herpesvirus simplex*; (2) *bacteria*, including *Listeria monocytogenes* and *Streptococcus pneumoniae*; and (3) *parasites*, including *Trichinella spiralis, Plasmodium benghei,* and *Schistosoma mansoni.*

A list of these and other infectious agents has been compiled by Bradley and Morahan (1982). Some details of the testing procedures and relevant references are provided in a number of recent papers (Dean et al., 1982a; Kerkvliet et al., 1982; Kern, 1982; Loose, 1982).

Cell-Mediated Immunity

This can be studied in intact animals or with cells in vitro. In the intact animals, usually mice, the commonly used procedure is to determine the delayed hypersensitivity response to a specific antigen. The antigen, such as sheep erythrocytes or keyhole limpet hemocyanin, is injected into a footpad or an ear of the animal. Four days later, a challenging dose of the antigen is given at the sensitized site. The extent of the swelling or the amount of localized radioactivity from a radiolabeled substance, e.g., ^{125}I-labeled human serum albumin or tritiated thymidine, is measured (Luster et al., 1982; Munson et al., 1982; Sanders et al., 1982).

In vitro tests are conducted on cells collected from animals pretreated with the test chemical. Such tests include lymphocyte proliferation and lymphocyte subpopulation.

The lymphocyte proliferation assay is done by culturing, in the presence of mitogens, lymphocytes collected from the spleen of pretreated animals. Mitogens such as phytohemagglutinin and concanavalin A are capable of inducing proliferation of normal T lymphocytes, whereas lipopolysaccharides, e.g., cell membrane of gram-negative bacteria, affect B lymphocytes. Immunosuppressive agents inhibit lymphocyte proliferation. The extent of proliferation can be determined by the incorporation of tritiated thymidine into DNA (Luster et al., 1982).

Lymphocytes, as noted above, consist of T cells, B cells, and null cells, and the T-cell population is composed of T-memory, T-helper, T-suppressor, and T-killer cells. Techniques for their enumeration include the use of immunofluorescence, rosette formation, histochemistry, cell electrophoresis, cytolysis, and fluorescence-activated cell sorting (Norbury, 1982).

Humoral Immunity

A commonly used procedure, the plaque assay, involves quantitative determination of plaque-forming cells (PFC) of the IgM class. Four days after the mouse has been sensitized to an antigen (e.g., sheep erythrocytes), the spleen is removed and a cell suspension is made. A quantity of the antigen, along with a suitable complement, is added to the suspension. The mixture is then spread on a slide and the number of plaques is counted. This represents the primary humoral immune response. To determine the secondary immune response, the mouse is given on day 10 a second dose of the antigen. On day 15 the spleen is removed and the above procedure is repeated with an additional step of incubation with rabbit anti-mouse IgG to develop the IgG-producing plaques. Reduced plaques indicate immunosuppression (Spyker-Cranmer et al., 1982). Instead of sheep erythrocytes, which are T-dependent antigens, lipopolysaccharides, which are T-independent antigens, may be used.

The levels of various immunoglobulins (IgG, IgM, IgA) in the serum may be directly measured. The techniques for there measurement have been reviewed by Davis and Ho (1976). The number of B cells in the spleen also provides information on the status of humoral immunity (Dean et al., 1982a). The procedures and advantages of the enzyme-linked immunosorbent assay (ELISA) in testing chemicals for immunotoxicity have been elaborated by Vos et al. (1982).

Macrophage and Bone Marrow

The functions of macrophages can be tested in a number of ways: (1) the number of resident peritoneal cells, (2) phagocytosis, (3) lysosomal enzymes, (4) cytostasis of tumor target cells, and (5) reticuloendothelial system uptake of ^{132}I-triolein. Parameters of bone marrow activity include (1) cellularity, (2) colony-forming units of multipotent cells, (3) colony-forming units of granulocyte/macrophage progenitors, and (4) iron incorporation in the bone marrow and spleen (Dean et al., 1982a).

Others

A variety of pathotoxicologic data may also be useful indicators of immune function: (1) hematology profile—hemoglobin, erythrocyte count, leukocyte count, differential cell count; (2) clinical chemistry—creatine phosphokinase (CPK), α-HBDH, SGPT, BUN, creatinine, acid and alkaline phosphatase, lactic dehydrogenase (LDH), cholinesterase; (3) serum proteins—albumin, globulin, albumin/globulin ratio; (4) weights—body, spleen, thymus, liver, kidney; and (5) histology—liver, thymus, adrenal, lung, kidney, heart, spleen (Dean et al., 1982a).

For example, thymic atrophy appears to be a very sensitive indicator of immunotoxicity. A paucity of lymphoid follicles and germinal centers in the spleen is indicative of B-cell deficiency, whereas T-cell deficiency is characterized by lymphoid hypoplasia in the paracortical areas.

REFERENCES

Adams, H. R., Parker, J. L., and Durrett, L. R. (1978) Cardiac toxicity of antibiotics. *Environ. Health Perspect.* 26:217–223.

Allmark, M. G., Grice, H. C., and Lu, F. C. (1955) Chronic toxicity studies on food colors: Observations on the toxicity of FD&C yellow No. 3 (Oil Yellow AB) and FD&C Yellow No. 4 (Oil Yellow OB) in rats. *J. Pharm. Pharmacol.* 7:591–603.

Aviado, D. M. (1978) Effects of fluorocarbons, chlorinated solvents, and inosine on the cardiopulmonary system. *Environ. Health Perspect.* 26:207–216.

Balazs, T., and Ferrans, V. J. (1978) Cardiac lesions induced by chemicals. *Environ. Health Perspect.* 26:181–191.

Balazs, T., Ferrans, V. J., et al. (1981) Study of the mechanism of hydralazine-induced myocardial necrosis in the rat. *Toxicol. Appl. Pharmacol.* 59:524–534.

Bardin, C. W., Baker, H. W. G., Jefferson, L. S., and Santen, R. J. (1978) Methods for perfusing male reproductive tract: Models for studying drugs and hormone metabolism. *Environ. Health Persect.* 24:51–59.

Brackett, B. G. (1978) In vitro fertilization: A potential means for toxicity testing. *Environ. Health Perspect.* 24:65–71.

Bradley, S. G., and Morahan, P. S. (1982) Approaches to assessing host resistance. *Environ. Health Persect.* 43:61–69.

Brusick, D. (1980) *Principles of Genetic Toxicology.* New York: Plenum Press.

Cohen, S., and McCluskey, R. T. (1979) Delayed hypersensitivity. In: *Principles of Immunology.* Eds. N. R. Rose, F. Milgrom, and C. J. van Oss. New York: Macmillan.

Davis, N. C., and Ho, M. (1976) Quantitation of immunoglobulins. In: *Manual of Clinical Immunology.* Eds. N. R. Rose and H. Friedman: Washington, D.C.: American Society of Microbiology.

Dean, J. H., Padanathsingh, M. L., and Jerrells, T. R. (1979) Assessment of immunological effects induced by chemicals, drugs or food additives. I. Tier testing and screening approach. *Drug Chem. Toxicol.* 2:5–17.

Dean, J. H., Luster, M. I., Boorman, G. A., and Lauer, L. D. (1982a) Procedure available to examine the immunotoxicity of chemicals and drugs. *Pharmacol. Rev.* 34:137–148.

Dean, J. H., Luster, M. I., Boorman, G. A., Luebke, R. W., and Lauer, L. D. (1982b) Application of tumor, bacterial and parasite susceptibility assays to study immune alterations induced by environmental chemicals. *Environ. Health Perspect.* 43:81–88.

Dixon, R. L. (1980) Toxic responses of the reproductive system. In: *Casarett and Doull's Toxicology.* Eds. J. Doull, C. D. Klaassen, and M. O. Amdur. Washington, D.C.: Hemisphere.

Eliasson, R. (1978) Semen analysis. *Environ. Health Perspect.* 24:81–85.

EPA (1982) *Health Effects Test Guidelines.* Washington, D.C.: U.S. Environmental Protection Agency.

Fabro, S. (1978) Penetration of chemicals into the oocyte, uterine fluid and preimplantation blastocyst. *Environ. Health Perspect.* 24:25–29.

Grice, H. C. (1972) The changing role of pathology in modern safety evaluation. *CRC Crit. Rev. Toxicol.* 1:119–152.

Jones, G. (1981) Toxicity requirements of the UK and EEC. In: *Testing for Toxicity.* Ed. W. Gorrod. London: Taylor & Francis.

Kerkvliet, N. I., Beecher-Steppan, L., and Schmitz, J. A. (1982) Immunotoxicity of pentachlorophenol (PCP); Increased susceptibility to tumor growth in adult mice fed technical PCP-contaminated diets. *Toxicol. Appl. Pharmacol.* 62:55–64.

Kern, E. R. (1982) Use of viral infections in animal models to assess changes in the immune system. *Environ. Health Perspect.* 43:71–79.

Lee, I. P., and Dixon, R. L. (1978) Factors influencing reproduction and genetic toxic effects on male gonads. *Environ. Health Perspect.* 24:117–127.

Lee, R. J., Zaidi, I. H., and Baky, S. H. (1978) Pathophysiology of the atherosclerotic rabbit. *Environ. Health Perspect.* 26:225–231.

Loose, L. D. (1982) Macrophage induction of T-suppressor cells in pesticide-exposed and protozoan-infected mice. *Environ. Health Perspect.* 43:89–97.

Luster, M. I., Dean, J. H., and Boorman, G. A. (1982) Cell-mediated immunity and its application in toxicology. *Environ. Health Perspect.* 43:31–36.

Merin, R. G. (1978) Myocardial metabolism for the toxicologist. *Environ. Health Perspect.* 26:167–174.

Morin, Y., and Daniel, P. (1967) Quebec beer-drinkers cardiomyopathy: Etiological considerations. *J. Can. Med. Assoc.* 97:926–931.

Morton, D. M. (1981) Requirements for the toxicological testing of drugs in the USA, Canada and Japan. In: *Testing for Toxicity*. Ed. W. Gorrod. London: Taylor & Francis.

Munson, A. E., et al. (1982) In vivo assessment of immunotoxicity. *Environ. Health Perspect.* 43:41–52.

Nagi, S., and Virgo, B. B. (1982) The effects of spironolactone on reproductive functions in female rats and mice. *Toxicol. Appl. Pharmacol.* 66:221–228.

Norbury, K. C. (1982) Immunotoxicology in the pharmaceutical industry. *Environ. Health Perspect.* 43:53–59.

Palmer, A. K. (1976) Assessment of current test procedures. *Environ. Health Perspect.* 18:97–104.

Sanders, V. M., et al. (1982) Humoral and cell-mediated immune status in mice exposed to trichloroethylene in the drinking water. *Toxicol. Appl. Pharmacol.* 62:358–368.

Sperelakis, N. (1978) Cultured heart cell reaggregate model for studying cardiac toxicology. *Environ. Health Perspect.* 26:243–267.

Spyker-Cranmer, J. M., Barnett, J. B., Avery, D. L., and Cranmer, M. F. (1982) Immunoteratology of chlordane: Cell-mediated and humoral immune responses in adult mice exposed *in utero*. *Toxicol. Appl. Pharmacol.* 62:402–408.

Stutman, O., Lattime, E. C., and Figarella, E. F. (1981) Natural cytotoxic cells against solid tumors in mice: A comparison with natural killer cells. *Fed. Proc.* 40:2699–2704.

Toy, P. A., Van Stee, E. W., Harris, A. M., Horton, M. L., and Back, K. C. (1976) The effects of three halogenated alkanes on excitation and contraction in the isolated, perfursed rabbit heart. *Toxicol. Appl. Pharmacol.* 38:7–17.

Van Stee, E. W. (1980) Myocardial toxicity. In: *The Scientific Basis of Toxicity Assessment*. Ed. H. R. Witschi. New York: Elsevier/North Holland.

Vos, J. G., Krajnac, E. I., and Beekhof, P. (1982) Use of the enzyme-linked immunosorbent assay (ELISA) in immunotoxicity testing. *Environ. Health Perspect.* 43:115–121.

Index